Schizophrenia

Peter B Jones MSc, PhD, FRCP, MRCPsych
Professor of Psychiatry
University of Cambridge
Cambridge, UK

Peter F Buckley MD, MRCPsych
Professor and Chairman
Department of Psychiatry and Health Behaviour
Medical College of Georgia
Augusta, Georgia, USA

With contributions by

David Kessler MD, MB BS, MRCPsych, MRCGP
General Practitioner
Senior Research Fellow in Department of
Community-Based Medicine
University of Bristol
Bristol, UK

CHURCHILL
LIVINGSTONE

ELSEVIER

D1057720

CHURCHILL
LIVINGSTONE
ELSEVIER

First published 2006.

ISBN 0443 102503

British Library Cataloguing in Publication Data
A catalogue record for this book is available from the British Library.

Library of Congress Cataloging in Publication Data
A catalog record for this book is available from the Library of Congress.

Notice
Knowledge and best practice in this field are constantly changing. As new research
and experience broaden our knowledge, changes in practice, treatment and drug
therapy may become necessary or appropriate. Readers are advised to check the most
current information provided (i) on procedures featured or (ii) by the manufacturer of
each product to be administered, to verify the recommended dose or formula, the
method and duration of administration, and contraindications. It is the responsibility
of the practitioner, relying on their own experience and knowledge of the patient, to
make diagnoses, to determine dosages and the best treatment for each individual
patient, and to take all appropriate safety precautions. To the fullest extent of the law,
neither the Publisher nor the Authors assume any liability for any injury and/or
damage to persons or property arising out or related to any use of the material
contained in this book.

The Publisher

Working together to grow
libraries in developing countries

www.elsevier.com | www.bookaid.org | www.sabre.org

ELSEVIER   BOOK AID International   Sabre Foundation

The
Publisher's
policy is to use
**paper manufactured
from sustainable forests**

Printed in Spain.

Contents

Preface

Schizophrenia is a debilitating and serious medical illness that has a profound effect on the patient's life, as well as the lives of their immediate family, friends and carers. The symptoms and course of the illness vary considerably between individuals, making diagnosis and subsequent management a complex task for the clinician.

Extensive research into the causes of schizophrenia and its treatment outcomes has resulted in a rapid pace of knowledge growth. Consequently, advances in treatment options and management of the condition have been substantial in recent years.

This book, jointly written by two experienced researchers and clinicians, aims to bring together all the latest research and current best practice in one easy-reference handbook for the busy clinician. The book is written concisely, with accompanying full-colour illustrations to help explain more difficult concepts. Case studies enable the reader to explore real-life patients and review their care plans with commentary from the authors. Finally, an excellent reference list allows the interested reader to gather further information on specific topics for themselves. The book is full of new information and clinical pearls, written in a condensed, pocket-book format.

We hope that this new book will be a valuable resource for the clinician and encourage a better understanding and appropriate management of schizophrenia patients.

Peter Jones
Professor of Psychiatry
University of Cambridge, Cambridge, UK

Peter Buckley
Professor and Chairman, Department of Psychiatry
Medical College of Georgia, Augusta, Georgia, USA

Biographies

Peter B Jones MB, MSc, MA, PhD, FRCP, MRCPsych, FMedSci is Professor of Psychiatry and Head of the Department of Psychiatry at the University of Cambridge. He read for his first degree in anatomy and neurobiology at King's College, London, before qualifying in medicine from Westminster Medical School. Following 3 years of general medical posts, Professor Jones began psychiatry at the Bethlem and Maudsley Hospitals in London where, after completing a masters degree in clinical epidemiology at the London School of Hygiene and Tropical Medicine and his PhD in psychiatric epidemiology, he was appointed as Senior Lecturer and Honorary Consultant Psychiatrist in 1993. In 1997 he took up the Chair of Psychiatry and Community Mental Health in Nottingham, moving to Cambridge in 2000.

Professor Jones' research concerns epidemiology of mental illness, particularly the psychoses, early lifecourse influences on adult mental health and illness, and the interface between population-based and biological investigations and explanations, including genetics. Clinically, he directs a new service for people with first episode psychosis (CAMEO, www.cameo.nhs.uk) jointly with Professor Ed Bullmore, and is presently a non-executive Director of the Cambridgeshire and Peterborough Mental Health Partnership NHS Trust.

Peter F Buckley, MD, MRCPsych is Professor and Chairman in the Department of Psychiatry at the Medical College of Georgia in Augusta. He immigrated to America in 1992 after completing his medical degree and post-doctoral training at the University College Dublin School of Medicine in Ireland. His thesis was on the subject of neuroimaging and neurodevelopment in schizophrenia.

Before joining the Department of Psychiatry at the Medical College of Georgia, Dr Buckley was Professor of Psychiatry and Vice Chair in the Department of Psychiatry at Case Western Reserve University School of Medicine in Cleveland, Ohio and served as Medical Director at Northcoast Behavioral Healthcare System (NBHS), the adult state psychiatric services for Cleveland and Toledo, Ohio.

Dr Buckley conducts research on the neurobiology and treatment of schizophrenia. He is author of a textbook on psychiatry and has edited eight specialist books on schizophrenia, as well as publishing widely in major psychiatric journals with over 250 book chapters, articles and abstracts. Dr Buckley is also Editor-in-Chief of the *Journal of Dual Diagnosis* and is on the editorial board of five other journals.

He is recipient of several awards for his work, including an Exemplary Psychiatrist Award from the National Alliance for the Mentally Ill. Dr Buckley is also the recipient of the 2004 American Psychiatric Association Administrative Psychiatric Award.

INTRODUCTION AND BACKGROUND

What is schizophrenia?

Schizophrenia is a collection of mental and behavioural phenomena, a clinical syndrome.[1] Its features may include: abnormal perceptions in the form of hallucinations; aberrant inferential judgements that result in extraordinary beliefs and delusions; distorted thought construction manifest as a disorder of language; unusual, often restricted, emotion, hedonia and volition; widespread cognitive problems particularly affecting memory and executive functions; seemingly strange behaviour explicable only in the context of these unusual experiences and deviant control systems; finally, it seems increasingly clear, as was known a century ago, that there are both motoric and developmental dimensions. This is quite a collection; no two cases are ever exactly the same.

Like many complex illnesses we know a lot about it in some senses, but many mysteries remain. Just under 1% of us experience the syndrome at some time in our lives, with a couple of dozen people per hundred thousand having a first onset each year. The schizophrenia syndrome is very rare indeed before puberty and most commonly has its onset in the first half of adult life. This must betray a lot about the underlying mechanisms of brain and mind, and the connectivity required to generate its features.

After a first episode, all outcomes are possible.[2] Some recover completely, many have a relapsing and remitting course for a decade or so, others experience a severe progressive, disabling disorder with premature death either from suicide or from a range of physical causes that are more common in people with the syndrome; lifestyle and common causes probably play a role in the latter. No single feature is either sufficient or necessary for the diagnosis, but many cases are obviously schizophrenia because a variety of characteristic features are present. Having said that, we are not sure where its edges are; there may be overlap with other mental illness such as affective or obsessive compulsive disorders, and there may be a spectrum of clinical abnormality that fades into a variety of exotic or unusual experiences in the general population.

We can treat schizophrenia and we know a lot about its genetic and environmental causes,[3] but we cannot cure it yet, neither do we have a decent classification of schizophrenia on the basis of causes, often seen as the pinnacle of nosology.[4] The disorder exists merely as a clinical syndrome of symptoms and signs that is generally useful and which is evolving.[5–7] We await a step-change in knowledge that will render this kind of definition out of date.

> *Schizophrenia is a collection of mental and behavioural phenomena, a clinical syndrome*

> *It seems increasingly clear that there are both motoric and developmental dimensions*

> *The schizophrenia syndrome most commonly has its onset in the first half of adult life. This must betray a lot about the underlying mechanisms of brain and mind, and the connectivity required to generate its features*

> *After a first episode, all outcomes are possible*

Fig. 1 DSM-IV: Schizophrenia.

Reprinted with permission from the *Diagnostic and Statistical Manual of Mental Disorder, Fourth Edition*, Text Revision. Copyright 2000 American Psychatric Association.[8]

Characteristic symptoms

Two (or more) of the following, each present for a significant portion of time during a 1-month period (or less if successfully treated):
- delusions
- hallucinations
- disorganized speech (e.g. frequent derailment or incoherence)
- grossly disorganized or catatonic behaviour
- negative symptoms, i.e. affective flattening, alogia or avolition

Note: Only one Criterion A symptom is required if delusions are bizarre or hallucinations consist of a voice keeping up a running commentary on the person's behaviour or thoughts, or two or more voices conversing with each other.

Social/occupational dysfunction

For a significant portion of the time since the onset of the disturbance, one or more major areas of functioning such as work, interpersonal relations or self-care are markedly below the level achieved prior to the onset (or when the onset is in childhood or adolescence, failure to achieve expected level of interpersonal, academic or occupational achievement).

Duration

Continuous signs of the disturbance persist for at least 6 months. This 6-month period must include at least 1 month of symptoms (or less if successfully treated) that meet Criterion A (i.e. active-phase symptoms) and may include periods of prodromal or residual symptoms. During these prodromal or residual periods, the signs of the disturbance may be manifested by only negative symptoms or two or more symptoms listed in Criterion A present in an attenuated form (e.g. odd beliefs, unusual perceptual experiences).

Schizoaffective and mood disorder exclusion

Schizoaffective disorder and mood disorder with psychotic features have been ruled out because either (1) no major depressive, manic or mixed episodes have occurred concurrently with the active-phase symptoms; or (2) if mood episodes have occurred during active-phase symptoms, their total duration has been brief relative to the duration of the active and residual periods.

Substance/general medical condition exclusion

The disturbance is not due to the direct physiological effects of a substance (e.g. a drug of abuse, a medication) or a general medical condition.

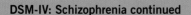

DSM-IV: Schizophrenia continued

Relationship to a pervasive developmental disorder

If there is a history of autistic disorder or another pervasive developmental disorder, the additional diagnosis of schizophrenia is made only if prominent delusions or hallucinations are also present for at least a month (or less if successfully treated).

Subtypes

295.20 Schizophrenia, Catatonic Type.
295.10 Schizophrenia, Disorganized Type.
295.30 Schizophrenia, Paranoid Type.
295.60 Schizophrenia, Residual Type.
295.90 Schizophrenia, Undifferentiated Type.

For a sufferer and their friends and family, then, schizophrenia can be a devastating and bewildering condition; for the clinician, it's a continuous and complex challenge, as well as being fascinating and puzzling from the social, biological and philosophical angles. Nevertheless, from a pragmatic point of view, when trying to help sufferers and their families, clinicians need reliable frameworks to give structure to their formulations, communicate and plan interventions and care. Operational criteria for the diagnosis of schizophrenia and related syndromes arose in the middle of the 20th century during an almost terminal bout of self-doubt in psychiatry, the pressures of the antipsychiatry movement and the contemporary requirements of health insurers. The fourth edition of the *Diagnostic and Statistical Manual* (DSM-IV)[8] and the *International Classification of Diseases*, 10th edition[9] are summaries of the most common, current, clinical ideas on the syndrome (see Figs 1 and 2). Work is beginning on new editions of both sets of criteria for schziophrenia, as well as on criteria for other mental illnesses.

Fig. 2 ICD-10: Schizophrenia (F20). Reproduced from *The ICD-10 Classification of Mental and Behavioural Disorders: Diagnostic Criteria for Research.* Geneva: WHO, 1993; pp. 64–65, with permission from the World Health Organization.

F20.0–F20.3 General criteria for paranoid, hebephrenic, catatonic and undifferentiated schizophrenia

G1 Either at least one of the syndromes, symptoms and signs listed under (1) below or at least two of the symptoms and signs listed under (2) should be present for most of the time during an episode of psychotic illness lasting for at least 1 month (or at some time during most of the days).

1 At least one of the following must be present:
- thought echo, thought insertion or withdrawal, or thought broadcasting;
- delusions of control, influence or passivity, clearly referred to body or limb movements or specific thoughts, actions or sensations; delusional perception;
- hallucinatory voices giving a running commentary on the patient's behaviour, or discussing the patient between themselves, or other types of hallucinatory voices coming from some part of the body;
- persistent delusions of other kinds that are culturally inappropriate and completely impossible (e.g. being able to control the weather, or being in communication with aliens from another world).

2 Or at least two of the following:
- persistent hallucinations in any modality, when occurring every day for at least 1 month, when accompanied by delusions (which may be fleeting or half-formed) without clear affective content, or when accompanied by persistent overvalued ideas;
- neologisms, breaks or interpolations in the train of thought, resulting in incoherence or irrelevant speech;
- catatonic behaviour, such as excitement, posturing or waxy flexibility, negativism, mutism and stupor;
- "negative" symptoms, such as marked apathy, paucity of speech and blunting or incongruity of emotional responses (it must be clear that these are not due to depression or to neuroleptic medication).

G2 Most commonly used exclusion clauses

If the patient also meets the criteria for manic episode (F30) or depressive episode (F32), the criteria listed under G1(1) and G1(2) above must have been met before the disturbance of mood developed. The disorder is not attributable to organic brain disease (in the sense of F00–F09) or to alcohol- or drug-related intoxication (F1x.0), dependence (F1x.2) or withdrawal (F1x.3 and F1x.4).

Subtypes

F20.1 Hebephrenic schizophrenia.
F20.2 Catatonic schizophrenia.
F20.3 Undifferentiated schizophrenia.
F20.4 Post-schizophrenic depression.
F20.5 Residual schizophrenia.
F20.6 Simple schizophrenia.
F20.8 Other schizophrenia.
F20.9 Schizophrenia unspecified.

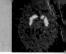

Presentation and natural history of schizophrenia

Diagnostic criteria show that the schizophrenia syndrome can have a variety of presentations; it can also run a variable course. This uncertainty about outcome leads commonly to problems in explaining what will happen to those with the syndrome and those who care for them. These problems limit the usefulness of schizophrenia as a diagnosis, and underpin the current habit of referring to the umbrella term of psychosis or non-affective psychosis to show that depression or mania are either not present or do not represent a better explanation for the illness. Psychosis is a less pejorative term and people may experience less stigma and be more accepting of the diagnosis themselves. It has its original roots in a very broad view of mental disturbance, but is now used to refer to specific symptoms or signs. Those who use the term psychosis need to be more specific about exactly what they mean, in terms of positive symptoms, negative features, social functioning, etc. They also need to understand the difference between classification, diagnosis, and a full clinical formulation and development of a care plan. People with these disorders are generally most keen on the last of these, with an interest in what will happen in the long term; classification is of far less interest to them.

We mentioned that the syndrome usually has an onset in early adult life, but the true beginning is often difficult to date. Schizophrenia is certainly a longitudinal concept, not merely a cross-sectional one. As will be seen from the section on antecedents, there are frequently differences in people who develop the syndrome noticeable from early life, albeit subtle. Thus, schizophrenia is something that develops over time. This means that it might be possible to do something about it sooner rather than later. Criteria such as the DSM-IV are couched in terms of an active phase of largely psychotic symptoms and a preceding, "prodromal" phase of less specific phenomena, that are obvious in retrospect, but don't add up to much when considered in terms of a diagnostic test. Certainly, the longer one is required to be ill before meeting criteria, the worse the outcome is likely to be.

The syndrome usually has an onset in early adult life, but the true beginning is often difficult to date

Features of the prodromal period include withdrawal from previous social roles, impairment in general functioning, behaviour others see as odd, altered emotions (blunted affect or inappropriateness), deterioration in personal hygiene, difficulties communicating with others, strange ideas, unusual perceptual experiences, and restricted drive, initiative, interests or energy.

These features are often summed up by others as the person "not being themselves"; people in a prodrome will sometimes say that "something is not quite right". The duration of the prodrome variable and its onset may be difficult to date. Sometimes, the onset is insidious

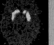

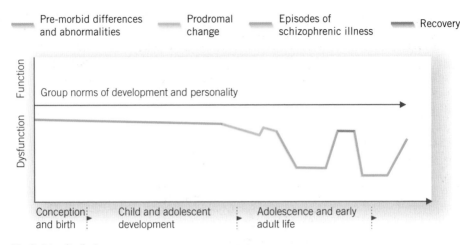

Fig. 3 **A longitudinal view of the evolution of schizophrenia**

and it may not be possible to identify a true change, particularly in younger people, who will be changing anyway as part of their normal development. In such cases, the loss of function and the more general concept of "social capital" can be profound. The prodome in these people will be developing just as they should be consolidating their education, occupational roles and adult relationships (Fig. 3).

One can see how the process of development of schizophrenia may evolve, and with it the diagnosis. One modern view of schizophrenia is that of an outcome of a process. There often appears to be continuity between pre-morbidly abnormal personality, insidious onset, disabling negative symptoms and poor outcome; some believe that this continuity is mediated by the cognitive deficits discussed later. However, the differential diagnosis of negative symptoms must always be borne in mind, because interventions that may be very effective differ (Fig. 4).

❝Even when there is a clear change, the prodrome is, despite its name, an entirely retrospective concept❞

Even when there is a clear change, the prodome is, despite its name, an entirely retrospective concept. We know definitely that a collection of suspicious and disabling features occur as a prodrome to schizophrenia once the schizophrenia syndrome has emerged, but there is much less certainty beforehand; features early in the prodrome may be very non-specific. As ever, we can be much more certain about the future after it has happened than before.

Early interventions

In addition to variability in the length of the prodrome, the length of time of active psychosis can vary greatly, commonly being measured in months or even years before people seek or get help. The reasons vary. This phase, or duration of untreated psychosis, is referred to as DUP.

Negative feature	Intervention
Depression	Antidepressant medication and psychological intervention such as cognitive therapy
Positive symptoms paradoxically leading to inactivity (e.g. running commentary hallucinations quelled only by inactivity)	Review antipsychotic drug regimen and consider cognitive or other psychological intervention
Extrapyramidal syndrome* thereafter	Review antipsychotic regimen, and be very careful
True negative symptoms	Review antipsychotic regimen and whole care plan, including occupational therapy and social aspects

*This may also be a feature at presentation; extrapyramidal features occur in drug-naive people.

Fig. 4 Differential diagnosis and management of apparent negative features

Neurobiological toxicity, with neural activity underlying psychosis strengthening neural networks – akin to *kindling*
Psychological trauma of frightening psychotic phenomena leading to features of post-traumatic stress disorder
Accrual of disabilities during untreated phase. The longer young people are ill, the further behind they fall in terms of education, occupation and social role development
Continuity of other factors such as abnormal pre-morbid personality, insidious onset, cognitive deficits and negative features. These drive poor outcome and, incidentally, lead to longer DUP

Fig. 5 Possible causes or mediators of long DUP and poor outcome

The length of the DUP does appear to be related to outcome; the longer the DUP, the worse the prognosis. The mechanism is not clear; there are several possible, or alternative, explanations (Fig. 5).

Further research is needed in order to decide which of these factors regarding DUP is most important, but it is possible that several or even all play a role. Certainly, many professional disciplines and most who use services can identify with one or several explanations. This may be helping to drive the expansion of specialist early intervention services aimed at first-episode psychosis, trying to reduce the DUP (Fig. 6); they are not necessarily aimed only at young people.

Clearly, it is important to identify people with psychosis as soon as possible after the onset of positive psychotic symptoms. A public health aim would, reasonably, be to identify people before they became psychotic, so long as there were interventions with an acceptable risk:benefit ratio. However, methods of prediction are as yet inadequate

Fig. 6 Interpretations of "early intervention" in psychosis

1. Before there is any sign of change or illness – primary prevention in the general population
2. Defining people at high risk but before there are overt signs of psychosis
3. Intervening in people with problems or *"At Risk Mental States"* who have made contact with services and, perhaps, are seen by a specialist service
4. Prompt, proper interventions for first-episode psychotic syndromes
5. Avoiding long delays in the delivery of effective intervention, care or rehabilitation in established schizophrenia

Fig. 7 Predictors of good outcome in schizophrenia

Female gender
Later age at onset – there is no threshold
Acute onset, often with apparent confusion
Precipitating factors or life events
Normal pre-psychotic personality
Good social, educational and occupational functioning
No negative features
No cognitive impairment
No family history of schizophrenia
Affective features or family history of affective disorder
Effective interventions maintained without side-effects
Not having the features of schizophrenia for long – a truism, but underlines the element of chronicity, and so poorer prognosis, built into the criteria

for this kind of screening to warrant the false positives; even careful follow-up would not necessarily be benign for these people who would, no doubt, be alarmed. Nevertheless, situations 3 and 4 in Fig. 6 are the proper remit of psychiatric services. Even if we cannot reliably identify prodromes without false positives, those who contact services with changed mental states are morbid and require help, regardless of whether they will develop psychosis. Trials in these situations are ongoing and important.[10] Situation 5 in Fig. 6 should now be obsolete in modern services. McGorry[11] has provided many excellent reviews of these issues and pioneering services in Australia.

Following an initial manic or psychotic syndrome, about 40% will never meet criteria for schizophrenia, having either long-term affective syndromes or non-affective diagnoses defined by their brief course, or their cause (such as drug intoxication).

For those who develop the schizophrenia syndrome, a residual or stable phase often follows the acute phase of the illness and the initiation of treatment. The features of this phase will often resemble the prodrome, frequently with some residual, attenuated psychotic phenomena that should be rigorously treated. However, emotional blunting or flattening and impairment in social role functioning is common.

The typical course is one of acute exacerbation, possibly precipitated by stress (but certainly stressful), illicit drug use, non-compliance with maintenance treatment, or a combination of these. There may be residual impairment between episodes. However, this course can be changed a great deal by the degree and quality of intervention provided, and is very variable between individuals.

Evidence from medium- and long-term follow-up from the WHO Ten Country Study[2,12] and elsewhere suggests that after 2–3 years this course will become clear, and that this may be a key period to get things right. Certainly, all concerned must remain optimistic during this initial period and focus efforts on making it more likely that the person concerned will have minimal residual symptoms or social impairment.

66After 2–3 years the course will become clear, and this may be a key period to get things right 99

Only some predictors of outcome are fixed (see Fig. 7). The nub of the early psychosis paradigm is to alter all malleable predictors, to engage people early in the assessment of their needs in a broad sense, to maximize the effectiveness of all interventions that are used, and to stick at it. The aim is to minimize impairment and promote recovery.

Social functioning and outcome

Schizophrenia involves impairment in many domains, often over and above the direct effect of positive psychotic features. Thus, one can describe a variety of disabilities that may affect someone with the disorder. The schema in Fig. 8 arose during the development of rehabilitation psychiatry, but remains useful if recent concepts are added.

Primary disabilities	• Positive and negative psychotic features • Depression and other psychopathology • Drug side-effects • Cognitive dysfunction
Secondary disabilities	• Loss of social capital • Education • Family • Friends • Occupational opportunity • Independence and esteem
Tertiary disabilities	• Results of stigma • Loss of opportunities • Discrimination

Fig. 8 Disabilities and impairments in schizophrenia – a conceptual framework

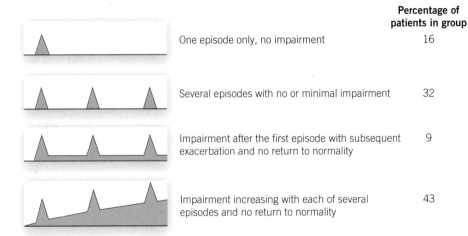

	Percentage of patients in group
One episode only, no impairment	16
Several episodes with no or minimal impairment	32
Impairment after the first episode with subsequent exacerbation and no return to normality	9
Impairment increasing with each of several episodes and no return to normality	43

Fig. 9 Five-year outcome following a first presentation of schizophrenia.
Services should aim to shift everyone up this caricature of outcome. Overall, we would hope to be doing somewhat better now than these figures indicate, but this shows the range of outcomes. Reproduced with permission of Cambridge University Press from *The Recognition and Management of Early Psychosis*, edited by McGorry PD, Jackson HJ, 1999. This was originally adapted from Shepherd M, et al. *Psychol Med* Monograph Suppl 1989;**15**:1–46.[13]

Impairments arise as a result of primary and, to some extent, tertiary disabilities (Fig. 9). They include occupational functioning, social relations and looking after oneself on a day-to-day level. This impairment varies across the different phases of the disorder, and is by no means always related to positive symptoms. Negative symptoms and cognitive problems are the key determinants, particularly when positive features are less potent for an individual, something that can be achieved with drug and psychological interventions, even when the phenomena themselves remain present. Certainly, they are more amenable to intervention than issues like society's attitudes to mental illness.

Some people may require supervision to ensure adequate nutrition and hygiene standards, and to protect the person from the consequences of impulsivity, poor judgement, cognitive impairment, or acting in response to delusional beliefs or command hallucinations. Between episodes of illness, the extent of residual disability may range from none to significant levels.

Violence by people with schizophrenia attracts media and public attention, and may influence health policy in a remarkably direct way. While the frequency of such acts is marginally higher than in the general population, this will be the same for many comparison groups and the absolute rates remain very low. The vagaries of normal human psychology, particularly in men, are responsible for a far greater toll of

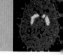

violence, and the risk in the population attributable to alcohol and other drug misuse is much higher than that attributable to any mental illness. The combination of positive features of schizophrenia, drug abuse and loss of contact with services and treatments is, however, a combination that does increase risk of violence,[14,15] that is amenable to treatment and that services should strive to avoid.

The life expectancy of people with schizophrenia is shorter than that of the general population. An important cause is suicide, with approximately 10% dying in this way; suicide prevention is another important aspect of any care plan. Accelerated mortality from a variety of other causes makes physical care and health promotion (including sexual health and drug advice) a vital consideration from first onset.

> *The combination of positive features of schizophrenia, drug abuse and loss of contact with services and treatments is, however, a combination that does increase risk of violence*

94 studies between 1960 and 1975. Heaton, Baade and Johnson, *Psychol Bull* 1978;**85**:141–62[16]
50% classification on the basis of neuropsychology is chance
For chronic schizophrenia (34 cases) there was only 54% correct classification – just about chance levels
Schizophrenia and brain damage appeared the same on the basis of neuropsychology in these studies during a period when some said schizophrenia was a myth

Fig. 10 Organic or functional? A comprehensive review of neuropsychological classifications of schizophrenic versus brain damaged

Cognition and neuropsychology

Kraepelin and Bleuler were both well versed in the experimental and cognitive psychology of their time, and emphasized underlying mechanisms in these spheres. The ideas went out of fashion in the middle of the 20th century, as psychodynamic formulations clouded the search for the causes of schizophrenia. Even so, as we have seen above, studies on general function, or IQ, were regularly showing a deficit in people with schizophrenia and, in fact, evidence of neuropsychological problems as severe as in acquired brain damage was present in the literature (see Fig. 10).

Over the past decade there has been a burgeoning of interest in neuropsychological deficits in schizophrenia, their relationship to symptoms and outcome, how they may map onto underlying neural systems, and how they may be manipulated (Fig. 11). This last issue is of particular interest, as there is substantial evidence for a strong link between neurocognitive deficits and poor functional outcome in schizophrenia (Fig. 12).[17] Interventions that could improve cognition would be helpful.

> *There is substantial evidence for a strong link between neurocognitive deficits and poor functional outcome in schizophrenia*

Fig. 11 What is the range of neuropsychological deficits?

Event-related potentials
Sustained attention • The Continous Performance Task
Selective attention
Memory • Explicit>implicit, recall and recognition • Working memory – dorsolateral prefrontal cortex (DLPFC)
Executive functions – planning and set-shifting
fMRI suggests less efficient frontal lobe function
General IQ one-third to one-half a standard deviation
Psychophysiology

Fig. 12 Neuropsychological mechanisms of psychosis and outcome are topical, and may represent the endo-phenotype in schizophrenia and other psychoses. They may also be the substrate upon which genetic risk has its action, amongst many other candidates. There may not be a single, vulnerable cognition or deficit, but a range of otherwise adaptive cognitive patterns may pose a risk of psychosis when they occur together. This is akin to genetic models involving multiple genes of small effect. Interested readers should consult a specialist reference. © Copyright 2005 Cambridge Cognition Limited. All rights reserved.

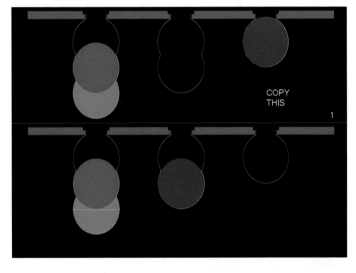

Attention, memory and executive functions are particularly implicated, with systems involving the dorsolateral prefrontal cortex important. It is likely that the continuity of abnormal pre-morbid personality, insidious onset, negative symptoms and poor outcome are all manifestations of the same underlying deficit. This may change with maturity of the relevant neural systems, perhaps reflecting genetic and epigenetic processes described later in the section on causes.

EPIDEMIOLOGY

Who gets schizophrenia?

Age

The safest answer is that anyone can get this syndrome. However, there are two remarkably constant findings in the epidemiology of schizophrenia. The first is that it tends to have its onset in young adulthood, being extremely rare before puberty. The figures from landmark studies by Slater and Cowie in the 1960s and by Häfner et al.[18] a quarter of a century later summarize the situation (Fig. 13) that has recently been extended and refined by Kirkbride and colleagues.[19] They also demonstrate the slight difference between men and women, who tend to have a somewhat later onset and longer period of risk. The close link between the life-course and the propensity to generate the schizophrenia syndrome probably betrays an underlying neurobiological phenomenon, such as the maturation of certain connections through normal or abnormal myelination.

66 Anyone can get this syndrome 99

66 Women tend to have a somewhat later onset and longer period of risk 99

Gender

The second consistent finding is that the disorder is rather more common in men when it is tightly defined in terms of excluding affective symptoms. Most studies with modern criteria include as few as half as many women as men in the first half of life, with the balance being restored later on. This increased incidence in women in later life, independently of dementia, may hold aetiological clues, with oestrogen systems implicated as protectors before the menopause.

66 The disorder is rather more common in men 99

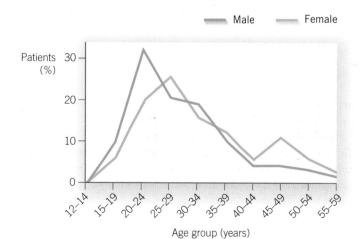

—— Male   —— Female

Patients (%)

Age group (years)

Fig. 13 Age at onset of schizophrenia.
Adapted from Häfner H, et al. *Br J Psychiat* 1993;**162**:80–6[18] with permission from the Royal College of Psychiatrists.

When does schizophrenia really begin?

The data on age at onset demonstrate that the emergence of the schizophrenia syndrome is intimately related to the life-course, and in an unusual way. In general, most pathological processes occur at the extremes of life, but schizophrenia occupies this intermediate position. This accounts, in part, for its huge personal, familial, social and economic impact.

Evidence of developmental differences is difficult to refine regarding those who will later become psychotic and those who will not. Kraepelin[20] and Bleuler[21,22] both noticed that a considerable proportion of people who developed the psychotic syndrome of schizophrenia had been different, in terms of character and behaviour, during childhood and youth.

> **"Kraepelin and Bleuler both noticed that a considerable proportion of people who developed the psychotic syndrome of schizophrenia had been different during childhood and youth"**

Their astute clinical observations were possible because they were, in large part, informally observing their patients' children before some developed illnesses similar to their parents. Thus, they made opportunistic use of genetic high-risk and cohort designs. However, the inference that the remainder of those who would develop schizophrenia had entirely *normal* development may not be justified.

Much of the evidence for abnormal development prior to psychosis, such as from studies of minor physical anomalies and neuropathology, is *best* (but not necessarily completely) explained in terms of developmental processes having gone wrong.[23] However, these processes are not observed directly. Genetic high-risk studies have shown subtle differences in neurological development in high-risk children.[24–27]

General population and genetic high-risk studies are two key tools. The evidence is convergent between the two research paradigms. General population cohorts can be considered as another type of high-risk paradigm where the children who will develop schizophrenia are at 100% risk, and are compared with their peers at zero risk.

High-risk studies

Developmental abnormalities throughout childhood have been found in one-quarter to one-half of "high-risk" children who are born to mothers with schizophrenia.[25,28] These include:

- hypoactivity;
- hypotonia and poor "cuddliness" during the neonatal period;
- an unusual pattern and slow attainment of milestones in infancy;
- "soft" neurological signs, in particular poor motor coordination in early childhood;
- deficits in attention and information processing in late childhood.

These findings indicate that at least part of the genetic vulnerability to schizophrenia involves, or is accompanied by, abnormal neurodevelopment. Attention and other cognitive deficits are likely to be of key importance.

Early milestones and motor development in general population studies

There is direct evidence of neurodevelopmental differences in children who will get schizophrenia as adults. Walker and Lewine[27] studied "home movies" of families in which one child later developed schizophrenia. They rated emotion and motor function blind to that child's identity amongst their siblings. The children who would as adults develop schizophrenia were distinguished on both accounts. Some remarkable, but transitory, motor differences were clear. Similar developmental differences have now been demonstrated in several epidemiological samples from around the world.

In the British 1946 birth cohort (the Medical Research Council National Survey of Health and Development, NSHD[29,30]), the first of the long-term, birth cohort studies in the UK, a range of childhood developmental differences were found.[31] Milestones were assessed by maternal recall at age 24 months, and all those recorded, sitting, standing, walking and talking, were delayed. There were indications that language development was different in these children. Health visitors were more likely to notice no speech by 2 years in the children who developed schizophrenia as adults, and school doctors noted speech delays and problems throughout childhood.

These developmental differences have been replicated in other cohorts. The British 1958 cohort (the National Child Development Study, NCDS) is the second of the three British birth cohorts and involves all children born in the same week as the NSHD, but 12 years later. Pre-schizophrenia children at age 7 had been slower to develop continence, and had poor coordination and vision. At age 16 they were rated clumsy.[32,33]

Cannon et al.[34] studied a cohort of births in Helsinki between 1951 and 1960, linking birth and school records to the Finnish Hospital Discharge Register. Children who had schizophrenia as adults were rated at school as having problems with sports and handicrafts. This may be a manifestation of the same uncoordinated motor characteristics as Crow et al.[32] demonstrated, and of the delayed milestones noted in the earlier British cohort.[35]

Two recent studies leave the existence of these subtle developmental abnormalities beyond doubt. The North Finland 1966 birth cohort

> *"These findings indicate that at least part of the genetic vulnerability to schizophrenia involves, or is accompanied by, abnormal neurodevelopment. Attention and other cognitive deficits are likely to be of key importance"*

66 Those who would later develop schizophrenia may have been walking just a little later than they might have been had they not have been subject to some pathological process that increased the risk of schizophrenia 99

66 These subtle effects have become one of the most replicated findings in the developmental epidemiology of schizophrenia 99

involved all 12,000 children due to be born in northern Finland during 1966.[36] Isohanni et al.[37] have indicated that the developmental differences are present even in the first year of life. There was evidence of a dose–response relationship between the age at which a boy could stand or walk without support, and his risk of subsequent schizophrenia; the later he walked, the more likely he was to develop schizophrenia (Fig. 14).

Not walking unsupported at age 1 is by no means abnormal, the absolute size of these effects is small, and schizophrenia is not solely a disorder of motor development. However, a dose–response relationship is a very potent finding in epidemiology, and the important thing about this one is that it operates within the normal range. Subjects who would later develop schizophrenia may have been walking just a little later than they might have been had they not have been subject to some pathological process that increased the risk of schizophrenia. It is not helpful to consider those who were late walkers in terms of being well below the mean as being at particular, or different, risk compared with the rest of the children who developed schizophrenia.

The latest results regarding early maturational effects before schizophrenia come from the Dunedin birth cohort study, in which continuity between self-reported psychotic experiences in childhood and a fairly broad concept of schizophreniform disorder arising by the early twenties has been reported recently.[38] Cannon et al.[39] have demonstrated similarly widespread developmental delays in several modalities before schizophreniform disorder, these being rather specific to this disease category. Figure 15 shows this for an early measure of motor competency.

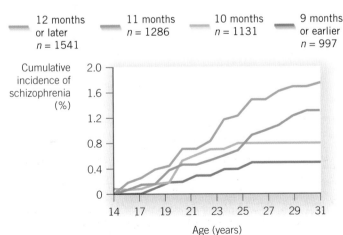

Fig. 14 The later a boy learned to stand during the first year of life, the greater was his risk of schizophrenia a decade or two later. Reproduced from Isohanni M, et al. *Schizophrenia Res* 2001;**52**:1–19[37] with permission from Elsevier.

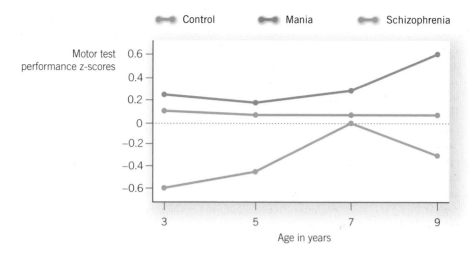

Fig. 15 **Mean standardized scores for motor development ages 3, 5 and 9 for adults diagnosed with schizophreniform disorder (*n* = 36) or mania (*n* = 20) compared with controls (*n* = 642).** Dunedin birth cohort. Adapted with permission from Cannon M, et al. *Arch Gen Psychiat* 2002;**59**(5): 449–56.[39] Copyright © 2002, American Medical Association. All rights reserved.

These subtle effects have become one of the most replicated findings in the developmental epidemiology of schizophrenia over the past decade. Each of the remarkable studies that have been investigated brings a slightly different view of the phenomenon. Regardless of their small size, these developmental differences are likely to betray biologically significant processes relevant to the development of schizophrenia (Fig. 16). They also indicate that causal processes were already active in very early life. It seems that the differences were most apparent "on the cusp" of developmental processes. Grown up, the children did not have gross motor or speech problems, although psychosis and the motor aspects of the schizophrenia syndrome[40] may be the later manifestations of the same mechanism(s), with the study by Poulton et al.[38] indicating hitherto unrecognized continuity of psychopathology. Kraepelin described motor problems in people with schizophrenia half a century before antipsychotic medication was described.

Later motor development milestones
More speech problems during childhood
Evidence of failure of integrative development and presence of soft signs
Lower educational test scores during childhood and adolescence
Preference for solitary play
Anxiety in social situations and sometimes problems with conduct

Fig. 16 **Summary of developmental differences prior to adult schizophrenia seen in the general population**

23

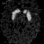

We are only just beginning to appreciate their significance, particularly as the frontostriatal systems that subserve motor development may be the same ones that are responsible for generating all or part of the schizophrenia syndrome later in life.[41]

> **"The frontostriatal systems that subserve motor development may be the same ones that are responsible for generating all or part of the schizophrenia syndrome later in life"**

Behavioural development

Studies of behaviour have also evolved from early clinical accounts. Retrospective assessment of behaviour and personality demonstrate differences prior to psychosis, with the most common being characteristics of a rather shy, schizoid habit.[42–45]

Robins[46] carried out a pioneering, historical cohort study in which she followed a group of boys who had been referred to a child guidance clinic. Antisocial behaviour was associated with later schizophrenia in this sample. Watt and Lubensky[47,48] traced the school records of cases of schizophrenia from a geographically defined neighbourhood in Massachusetts. Girls who were later to develop schizophrenia were introverted throughout kindergarten into adolescence. Boys in the same predicament were "disagreeable", but only in the later school grades (7–12). Done et al.[49] have identified a remarkably similar behavioural pattern in the British 1958 birth cohort, including the changes over time. "Schizoid" behavioural differences are seen in the British 1946 cohort,[50] and in two large studies of conscripts in Sweden[51] and Israel.[52,53]

Given current views (again re-learning what Kraepelin and Bleuler already thought) concerning the cognitive disturbances that accompany, and may underpin, psychosis, it seems a reasonable and parsimonious hypothesis that the early developmental and behavioural effects may be linked through cognition.[54] The motor and language findings betray a disturbance or difference in developmental processes. This is manifest in behavioural terms because the same processes affect cognitive development, particularly in the realm of social cognition. Any difference in behaviour and interaction with others may well, itself, lead to attenuation of social environment and further deviance in development through perturbation of the normal genetic, social–environmental and neurodevelopmental interactions that are involved in brain growth. This has been described as a "self-perpetuating cascade"[31] of abnormal development towards schizophrenia (Fig. 17).

> **"Any difference in behaviour and interaction with others may lead to attenuation of social environment and further deviance in development through perturbation of the normal genetic, social–environmental and neurodevelopmental interactions: a "self-perpetuating cascade" of abnormal development towards schizophrenia"**

Cognitive function and IQ before the schizophrenia syndrome

We have already noted that specific and general cognitive functions are abnormal in schizophrenia. Studies of pre-psychotic personality have largely confirmed the earliest clinical accounts; investigation of pre-

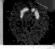

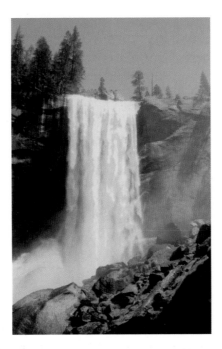

Fig. 17 Development prior to psychosis may be like a cascade, with some events and experiences early on determining the precise course thereafter, with an almost infinite number of routes to a particular place in the pool

psychotic IQ has challenged the initial notion of a deteriorating, dementing course after onset of psychosis, but the field remains controversial. Aylward et al.[55] have provided a comprehensive review of intelligence in schizophrenia. Standardized measures show intellectual function is lower in pre-psychotic individuals than in age-matched controls. Linking the pre-psychotic deficit to outcome, they raise the question as to whether IQ may be an independent factor that can protect otherwise vulnerable individuals, or whether the deficits are part of that vulnerability. Furthermore, we are not sure of what happens to this deficit over time.[56–60]

Albee et al.[61,62] compared childhood Stanford–Binet scores with Wecshler–Bellevue scores during adult schizophrenia psychosis in 112 people. Their longitudinal perspective allowed the authors to conclude that their results "seriously challenge the belief that intellectual loss occurs as a consequence of adult schizophrenia". Thirty-five years on, Russell et al.[63] have provided confirmatory evidence for this, but the effect remains controversial. In fact, the argument as to whether there is a developmental or degenerative process is probably a debate over a spurious dichotomy, given that a single, life-course process may be affected by a pathological process. Whether it's developmental or degenerative depends on the stage at which you begin to look at it. As

The argument as to whether there is a developmental or degenerative process is probably a debate over a spurious dichotomy, given that a single, life-course process may be affected by a pathological process

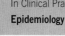
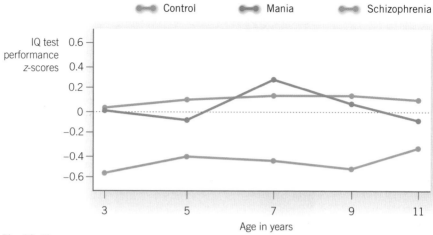

Fig. 18 **Mean standardized scores for intelligence tests at ages 3, 5, 7, 9 and 11 for adults diagnosed with schizophreniform disorder (*n* = 36) or mania (*n* = 20) compared with controls (*n* = 642).** Dunedin birth cohort. Adapted with permission from Cannon M, et al. *Arch Gen Psychiat* 2002; **59**(5):449–56.[39] Copyright © 2002, American Medical Association. All rights reserved.

shown in Fig. 18, taken from the Dunedin cohort,[39] the effect is certainly present in early life before schizophrenia, and may be specific to that disorder. In the 1946 British birth cohort (see above), several measures of educational achievement were collected on all children at ages 8, 11 and 15 years.[64,65] The data and results are summarized by Jones[66] and show tantalizing but statistically inconclusive evidence of decline during adolescence before schizophrenia (Figs 19 and 20).

Current interest in the cognitive aspects of schizophrenia[17,68] suggests a parsimonious conclusion that pre-psychotic IQ deficits (and perhaps social characteristics) may, indeed, be manifestations of the same abnormal cognitive processes that later result in psychosis, as was suggested earlier.

The relevance of the evidence that people who develop schizophrenia may have developmental differences before psychosis begins is of relevance to clinical practice, diagnosis and prevention (Fig. 21). Much more research on prediction and the specificity of these antecedent factors is required before these ideas are translated into services.[69,70]

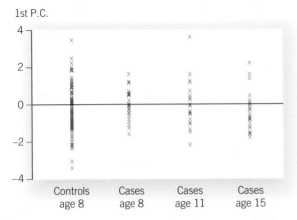

Fig. 19 IQ in children in the 1946 birth cohort comparing those who did not develop schizophrenia as adults (scores at age 8 years) and those who did (scores at ages 8, 11 and 15 years). Mean scores were lower, and there was no evidence of a threshold effect below or above which this relationship did not hold. Very bright individuals did develop schizophrenia, but they were much less likely than those who are less able. Put another way, any individual is more likely to develop schizophrenia than someone who is more able in terms of IQ, although the effect is small.

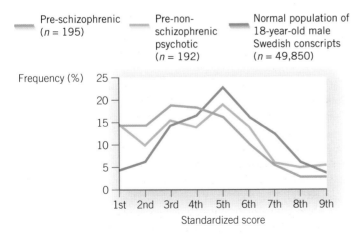

Fig. 20 The same kind of relationship between pre-psychotic IQ and later schizophrenia was shown in the Swedish conscript study. Here the measure was at age 18 and the left-shift consistent with a widespread effect is clear. Reproduced from David AS, et al. *Psychol Med* 1997;**27**(6): 1311–23[67] with permission from Cambridge University Press.

Fig. 21 Much research on the developmental antecedents of schizophrenia has had the study of causes as its focus. Results that people who will develop schizophrenia have pre-psychotic abnormalities may also have relevance for clinical work and even for prevention. There is a long way to go before we can use this approach routinely.

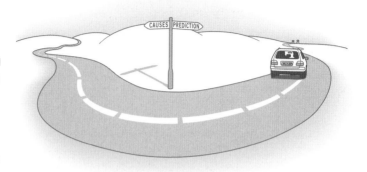

How many people have schizophrenia?
Prevalence data

How many people have schizophrenia at any one time? Two large studies of the prevalence of psychiatric disorders have been carried out in the USA that indicate a decrease in the prevalence of schizophrenia over one decade. Other major studies have been undertaken in Europe and Australia.

The Epidemiological Catchment Area programme[71] (ECA) surveyed 17,803 people between 1980 and 1984. This study indicated a lifetime prevalence of schizophrenia of 1.4%.[71] The National Comorbidity Survey[72] (NCS) interviewed 8098 people between 1990 and 1992 and found that lifetime prevalence for the summary category of non-affective psychosis was 0.7%.

The major prevalence study of psychiatric morbidity carried out in the UK, between April and September 1993 (OPCS), found a previous 6-month prevalence rate of only 0.4% for functional psychosis among people aged 16–64 living in private households.[73,74] This finding was very similar to the results from a large survey of psychotic disorders embedded within the Australian National Survey of Mental Health and Wellbeing,[75] where the weighted mean point prevalence for service contact was 4.7 per 1000 adults; over 60% of these people had schizophrenia or schizoaffective disorder (http://www.health.gov.au/hsdd/mentalhe/resources/reports/pdf/overview.pdf).

While being of the same order of magnitude, there are discrepancies between these estimates from different studies; even the seemingly simple question of prevalence cannot be answered definitively. Discrepancies may be related to issues of sampling or interview methodology. They remain to be clarified by future reports. However,

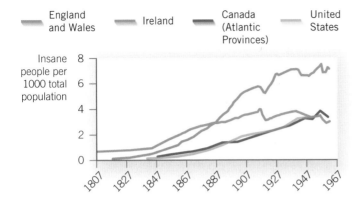

England and Wales	Ireland	Canada (Atlantic Provinces)	United States

Fig. 22 Counts of "insanity" rose in many parts of the West during the 19th century. Not all would have had schizophrenia, but the picture speaks for itself. Reprinted from Torrey EF, Miller J. *The Invisible Plague. The Rise of Mental Illness from 1750 to the Present.*[76] Copyright © 2001 by E Fuller Torrey and Judy Miller, with permission from Rutgers University Press.

at present, it seems that the lifetime prevalence of schizophrenia in the Western world may have decreased over the past decade. This could be due to lower incidence or changes in course that would include those secondary to better treatment.

Incidence data

Changes over time

The data suggest a roller-coaster: up and down they go. It seems clear that schizophrenia became more noticeable in the population in the late 18th century and throughout the 19th (Fig. 22). Whether this was due to a true increase in incidence, possibly due to new causes or greater prevalence of exposure to an old one, or to a change in the way society dealt with mental illness, is not clear. Both the late Edward Hare in the UK and, more recently, E Fuller Torrey in the USA[76] have written about this phenomenon extensively.

In the 20th century, the story has been one of apparent decline, then increase in a rather strange way that cannot have a single cause; the changes are dramatic (Fig. 23). Eagles and Whalley[78] were first to report a decline in the diagnosis of schizophrenia among first admissions in Scotland between 1969 and 1978. Since then, there have been 14 papers examining this issue in England, Scotland, Denmark, New Zealand, Canada, Ireland, the USA and the Netherlands (for a review, see Jones and Cannon[79]). In general, those based on national statistics have found a large (40–50%) decline in first admission rates for schizophrenia during the 1970s and the 1980s. However, findings based on case register data have been less consistent.

Fig. 23 First admission rates for schizophrenia and paranoia by sex and age. It was shown that rates of schizophrenia seemed to have fallen in the late 20th century, but they may have gone up again. Reproduced from Der G, et al. *Lancet* 1990;**335**:513–6[77] with permission from Elsevier.

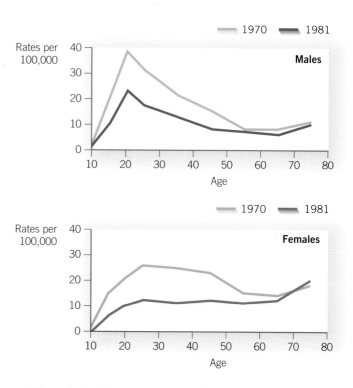

Hospital admission rates may be influenced by many factors, such as the introduction of more restrictive diagnostic criteria for schizophrenia, the move to community care, and changes in the age, sex and ethnic structure of the population. Has there really been a decrease?

66*Clinical experience suggests that the incidence is not decreasing*99

Clinical experience suggests that the incidence is not decreasing, certainly not so that health services would notice. Using incidence data from a large study of first service contacts for any psychosis in Nottingham, UK and comparing these with data from a previous census that formed part of the WHO Ten Country Study,[80] Brewin et al. have noted an increase in the incidence of all psychosis categories during the 1980s and early 1990s. This was not due to an increase in any particular diagnosis, such as drug-induced psychoses. Furthermore, a third study from this city at the end of the 1990s indicates that the trend continues, while a fourth[81] and a fifth[82] show similar effects in London and south-west Scotland, respectively, arguing strongly against the disappearance hypothesis, which has to be dead in the water.

Geographical variation

The largest, multi-centre study of the incidence of schizophrenia was initiated by the World Health Organization in the late 1970s.[83]

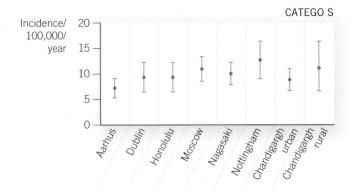

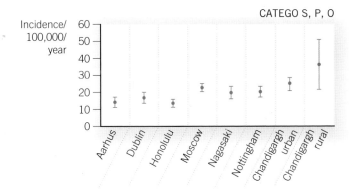

Fig. 24 Incidence data from WHO Ten Country Study. Adapted from Jones PB, Cannon M. Schizophrenia. In: Martyn CJ, Hughes RAC, editors. *The Epidemiology of Neurological Disorders.* London: BMJ Books, 1997[79] with permission from Blackwell Publishers.

Although there was little variation between the countries for narrowly defined schizophrenia (CATEGO "S") compared with broad (CATEGO "S, P and O"), the confidence estimates for the latter estimates were wide (Fig. 24). There may not have been enough power to detect considerable differences in the narrow definition,[79] and we are left not knowing whether the differences of about two-fold in broadly defined disorder are real or an artefact; the textbook point that schizophrenia occurs to a similar degree throughout the world is not really supported.

Incidence on other geographic levels – urban birth and migration
Schizophrenia and cities

The best evidence to date indicates that the incidence of schizophrenia is more common in people living in cities as compared with rural areas (Fig. 25); large studies from Denmark,[84,85] Finland,[86] the Netherlands,[87] the UK and elsewhere all show this. Moreover, it seems that the toxic period, if there is one, may be in early life.[88]

> **The incidence of schizophrenia is more common in people living in cities as compared with rural areas**

Fig. 25 Something about cities increases the risk of schizophrenia for those who live in them. M. C. Escher's "Convex and Concave". © 2005, The M. C. Escher Company – Holland. www.mcescher.com

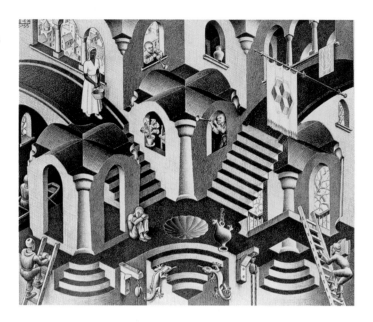

This urban finding is not new. Analysis from the 1880 US census by Torrey et al.[89] showed this phenomenon, as did the classic study in 1920s Chicago by the social scientists, Farris and Dunham. They exploited the concentric rings of social advantage and disadvantage in that city, where the inner area is the poorest and things improve towards the suburbs (Fig. 26). The figure shows that the incidence of schizophrenia estimated over 10 years is closely related to social advantage. Causation is another matter, although drift into cities by vulnerable or ill people has been shown not to account for this, particularly given the association with early life.

The same phenomenon was found three-quarters of a century later in the city of Nottingham in the UK by Croudace et al.[91] (Fig. 27). In this line of enquiry we are still not sure whether it is the "urbanicity", the social disadvantage or a combination of both these elusive concepts that is operating to modify risk. The phenomenon is also a good example of something clear in one research discipline (say, epidemiology) that is rather difficult to explain in another (say, psychopharmacology); that's why it's interesting! Many hypotheses have been put forward, some of the most popular being brain damage due to exposure to infectious agents and increased psychosocial stress acting as a trigger. Migration from other areas and countries may play a part, but this phenomenon, too, requires explanation.

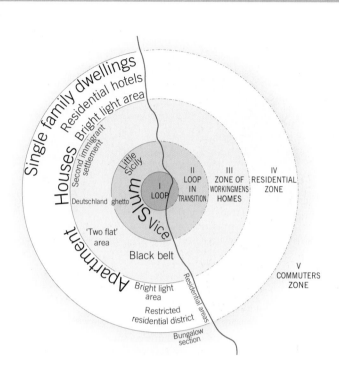

Fig. 26 Farris and Dunham's demonstration of a link between city life in Chicago and incident schizophrenia. Reproduced with permission from Faris R, Dunham HW. *Mental Disorders in Urban Areas*, 2nd ed. New York: Hafner Publishing, 1960.[90]

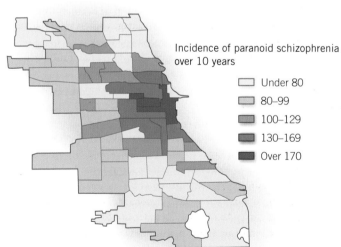

Incidence of paranoid schizophrenia over 10 years

☐ Under 80
☐ 80–99
☐ 100–129
☐ 130–169
■ Over 170

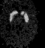

Fig. 27 The 2-year incidence of any psychotic illness in each electoral ward (about 4000 people) in Nottingham, UK, and the spatial association with socio-economic advantage measured with MINI, a scale summarizing a number of survey characteristics. High MINI scores indicate poorer areas. Incidence of psychosis can effectively be presented on the same colour scale, being most common in the deprived areas. The association between poorer areas and higher incidence of psychosis is clear, but not explained. Data from Croudace TJ, et al. *Psychol Med* 2000;**30**:177–85.[91]

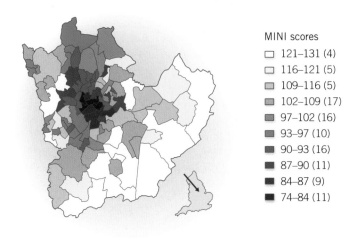

MINI scores
☐ 121–131 (4)
☐ 116–121 (5)
▨ 109–116 (5)
▨ 102–109 (17)
▨ 97–102 (16)
▨ 93–97 (10)
▨ 90–93 (16)
■ 87–90 (11)
■ 84–87 (9)
■ 74–84 (11)

Schizophrenia and immigration

Schizophrenia appears to be more common in some populations that have migrated. In 1988, the psychiatric community and beyond was surprised by a report that the incidence of schizophrenia among the African-Caribbean population in Nottingham was more than 1000% higher than in the general population.[80] Several replications from other centres in the UK[92–95] and in the Netherlands[96] confirm this effect, although the true incidence ratio is now thought to be rather lower (around five-fold) when the denominator is adjusted for possible under-reporting in census data and, perhaps, due to a period or cohort effect.[92,93] An increased incidence ratio for schizophrenia has also been found among African[92,93] and Asian[93] immigrants in the UK, indicating that the effect is not confined solely to a single ethnic minority; nor, indeed, is it confined to schizophrenia.[80] The hospital admission rate for schizophrenia among migrants is higher in their host country than in their country of origin,[97,98] implicating factors occurring principally after migration. The risk of schizophrenia appears greater for second-generation migrants than first-generation migrants,[94,95,99,100] arguing against selective migration of pre-schizophrenia individuals, as do the findings of Selten and Sijben.[96] The fact that immigrants from poor countries tend to show higher rates of schizophrenia than immigrants from affluent countries[101] implies that factors associated with improved living conditions, industrialization or urbanization may be involved. If we could only explain this phenomenon, we'd know a lot more about schizophrenia and its causes.

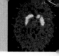

AETIOLOGY AND DIAGNOSIS

What causes schizophrenia?

The foregoing epidemiology gives many clues to causes. It is becoming clear that most diseases are neither purely genetic nor purely environmental in origin, but depend on a complex interaction of the two.[102,103] Twin studies are a powerful way of investigating this (Fig. 28).

As the figure suggests, schizophrenia is likely to be no exception; twin studies clearly demonstrate this. Monozygotic twins share 100% of their genes, but when one monozygotic twin has schizophrenia, up to 50% of their co-twins are unaffected. Such studies clearly point to the importance of environmental factors in the aetiology of the disorder.[105] This seemingly clear logic was lost in the mid-20th century, but we are on firmer ground again now, even if we do not yet have all the answers.

When we ask "What causes schizophrenia?", Jones and Cannon[79] defined three aspects:

- What are the genes contributing to the causation of schizophrenia, where are they located, when are they expressed and for what proteins do they code?
- What environmental factors are involved in the causation of schizophrenia and when do they have their effects?
- How do the genetic and environmental factors interact with each other?

Does schizophrenia run in families?

Schizophrenia does run in families, but by no means everyone with schizophrenia has an affected relative;[106] this figure is said to be about 80% but can go down if a careful history is taken. In general,

Most diseases are neither purely genetic nor purely environmental in origin, but depend on a complex interaction of the two

Schizophrenia does run in families, but by no means everyone with schizophrenia has an affected relative

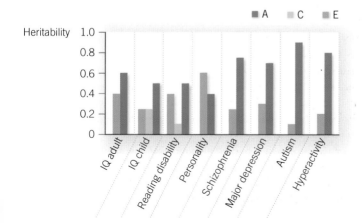

Fig. 28 Estimates of genetic and environmental effects from recent twin studies. A, additive genetic variance, or heritability; C, variance from shared environment; E, variance resulting from non-shared environment and measurement errors. Data from Plomin R, et al. *Behavioural Genetics.* New York: Freeman, 2001.[104]

35

Fig. 29
Schizophrenia does show familiality that is genetic, but currently there is no evidence that pushing a genetic button leads inexorably to schizophrenia. The pathway is complex.

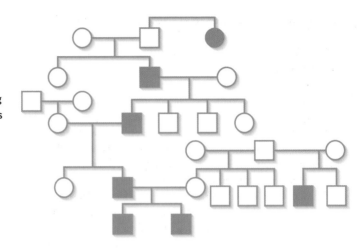

the first-degree relatives of people with schizophrenia (though this is a matter of debate of late) have a 3–7% risk for schizophrenia, 5–10-fold higher than that found in relatives of general population controls. This excess risk of schizophrenia occurs predominantly among the children and siblings of people with schizophrenia. Parents are at lowest risk; the adverse effects on fertility associated with the condition mean that parents tend to be "selected for health" and have already survived much of the period of risk (Fig. 29).[107,108]

Familiality of a disease does not necessarily imply a genetic causation. Twin and adoption studies are needed to determine to what extent the familial aggregation is due to genetic versus environmental factors.

Adoption studies

Adoption studies can tease apart the effect of family environment or styles of bringing up children from the effect of the genetic constitution of the children or parents.

The Copenhagen adoption study established a genetic basis to the familial aggregation of schizophrenia.[109,110] The results show an increased risk of schizophrenia in the biological relatives of adoptees from parents with schizophrenia, but not in the adoptive relatives or in control adoptees. Results have been similar from a large adoption study in Finland.[111,112]

An increased risk of schizophrenia in the absence of any contact with biological relatives indicates that genetic factors are important or necessary. Of course, this does not rule out the possibility of gene–environment interactions. Furthermore, the adopted child has still spent the prenatal period with the biological mother. However, in the Danish adoption study, the risk of schizophrenia spectrum disorders was also increased in the paternal half-siblings of the adoptee of relatives with schizophrenia that shared neither the prenatal nor the familial environment.[108]

Twin studies

Twelve major twin studies of schizophrenia have been carried out. They all show that the risk for schizophrenia in the co-twin of a schizophrenia proband (the probandwise concordance) is substantially higher for monozygotic (MZ; 53%) than dizygotic (DZ; 15%) twins,[106] giving an overall heritability estimate of 68% for the underlying liability to schizophrenia. Recent results from an epidemiological twin study of schizophrenia in Finland using model fitting indicate that 83% of the variance in liability to schizophrenia is due to additive genetic factors and the remaining 17% is due to unique environmental factors, with no effect for shared environment.[34] MZ discordance for schizophrenia may be caused by the "reduced penetrance" of a schizophrenia genotype, or the presence of "sporadic" or non-genetic cases. The first, but not the second, explanation would predict an increased risk of schizophrenia among the offspring of the unaffected twin of a discordant MZ pair, which has been upheld in a study by Gottesman and Bertelsen.[113] This suggests that environmental factors alone are seldom sufficient to cause schizophrenia, though they may play a decisive role in some individuals genetically predisposed to schizophrenia.

What are the genes doing?

One can think of this in two ways, in a molecular sense or in a psychological sense. Jones and Murray[114] noted that "genes code for proteins, not for delusions or hallucinations", and suggested a range of target molecules that might be involved in relevant developmental processes. Recent advances in functional genomics and proteomics are likely to take this logic forward. However, the psychological approach remains important and relevant.

"Genes code for proteins, not for delusions or hallucinations"

Schizotypy

We have already mentioned the idea of a neuropsychological endophenotype, but there may also be a behavioural one that can be present without the schizophrenia syndrome. Family, twin and adoptive studies all show that certain psychiatric illnesses and personality disorders, known as the "schizophrenia spectrum", are genetically allied to schizophrenia.[115]

The most important of these disorders appears to be schizotypal personality disorder (SPD) (Fig. 30). The relative risk for SPD in the

Fig. 30 DSM-III-R diagnostic criteria for schizotypal personality disorder. Reprinted with permission from the *Diagnostic and Statistical Manual of Mental Disorder, Fourth Edition,* Text Revision. Copyright 2000 American Psychatric Association.[8]

Odd communication
Inadequate rapport in face-to-face interaction
Magical thinking
Ideas of reference
Suspiciousness
Recurrent illusions
Social isolation
Undue social anxiety or hypersensitivity to criticism
Odd or eccentric behaviour

first-degree relatives of schizophrenia probands compared with controls is about five-fold.[107,116] Parents of people with schizophrenia have a higher risk of SPD than siblings, suggesting that individuals who inherit this "milder" genetic vulnerability are responsible for the maintenance of schizophrenia in the population.[117]

Uncertain validity and the lack of biological markers apply to SPD as much, if not more, than to schizophrenia itself. Many scales have been developed to diagnose SPD and measure "schizotypy",[118] usually self-administered questionnaires.

The major disadvantage is that the aspects of the diagnosis of SPD, which are most "predictive" of having a relative with schizophrenia, are the most subjective:[119] odd speech patterns, negative symptoms (aloofness/poor rapport), social dysfunction and avoidant symptoms, all factors that discourage participation in research. The most promising line of enquiry for diagnosis of SPD is detailed interview with all relatives of schizophrenia patients, particularly siblings, but this will be difficult to achieve.

The study of the siblings of people with schizophrenia is becoming increasingly popular in the field of neuropsychology.[120] Many siblings show neuropsychological abnormalities that are intermediate between the abnormalities shown by the patients and the performance of normal controls, linking these lines of psychology and personality.

The "schizophrenia spectrum"

Other disorders which form part of the "schizophrenia spectrum" are schizoaffective disorder,[108] paranoid personality disorder[117] and schizoid personality disorder,[109,116] although there is some debate about the last of these.[117] No excess of anxiety disorder or alcoholism has been found in the relatives of schizophrenia patients compared with the relatives of controls, indicating that the genetic transmission of schizophrenia and schizophrenia spectrum disorders is relatively specific, and does not include a generalized liability to all psychiatric illness.[109,116,121] The debate about whether affective disorders occur to excess in the relatives of schizophrenia patients has not yet been resolved.[121–123] Relatives of schizophrenia patients do appear to have an increased predisposition to develop psychotic symptoms as part of an affective illness.[121] It may be that psychosis, or a vulnerability to it, is inherited, with other factors acting in a pathoplastic manner.

A "continuum" approach to measurement of schizophrenia

The "schizophrenia spectrum" has been talked about for many years, although little hard evidence for its existence has existed until recently. The notion of a "schizophrenia continuum" may be a more useful way to conceptualize the relationship between schizophrenia and these other disorders, particularly schizotypal personality disorder. The progression of schizotypal features into frank schizophrenia has been demonstrated,[124] though not definitively. It is also known that schizophrenia itself has a much wider range of outcome and prognoses than previously thought, with about half of patients showing "good social adjustment at follow-up" and about 20% showing almost complete recovery after one episode.[79] Few accept that a neat, categorical approach to schizophrenia is going to illuminate the truth, and some, such as Crow and Liddle, have applied different dimensional models to causation and to symptoms, respectively.

Genetic models

The true mode of inheritance is likely to be "complex".[125] Risch[126] has shown that the pattern of recurrence risks in relatives of schizophrenia probands is inconsistent with a single locus and several genome scans have now excluded this. The generally accepted aetiological model for schizophrenia is a combination of multiple genes and environmental factors.[115] The model has also been regarded as a liability/threshold model, with total liability above a certain value being equivalent to disease.[7,105] On simple additive models, it is generally agreed that roughly 70% of the variation in the liability in the general population is attributable to genetic variation among individuals (Fig. 31). However, this tells us little about the nature of the genetic contributions, the environmental contributions, or their interactive contributions to the risk for schizophrenia.[127]

Fig. 31 How the hand of genetic cards in some families means that more pass the threshold of risk or disorder than compared with the population average

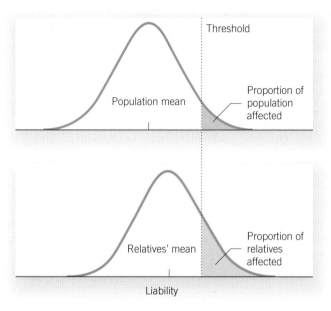

The search for susceptibility genes for schizophrenia and quantitative traits

Genes that contribute to genetic variance in quantitative traits are known as quantitative trait loci (QTL).[128] Both linkage and association methods have been developed to map QTLs in humans (Fig. 32). Another QTL approach is the use of a continuous outcome measure that is biologically related to schizophrenia, such as schizotypy.[130]

Linkage studies

Linkage analysis assesses the association of markers and alleles within families (Fig. 33). Two common approaches are the traditional lod score approach and the more recent affected-relative-pair approach. Both have been used in the study of schizophrenia, but the latter is preferable because it does not require the mode of inheritance to be specified.[115] Further issues regarding variance and causation are reviewed by Lewontin.[131]

The Schizophrenia Linkage Collaborative Group[132] was designed to follow up on three previously published positive findings resulting from large-scale genome scans by individual groups: the 6p finding of Straub et al.[133] and the 3p and 8p findings of Pulver et al.[134] This study obtained support (but certainly not "proof") for the hypotheses that loci on chromosomes 6 and 8 have genetic variation involved in determining the level of susceptibility to schizophrenia; the data do seem to

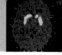

Gene	Locus	Strength of evidence (0 to +++++) for			
		Assoc. with schizophrenia	Linkage to gene locus	Biological plausibility	Altered expression in schizophrenia
COMT	22q11	++++	++++	++++	Yes, +
DTNBP1	6p22	+++++	++++	++	Yes, ++
NRG1	8p12–21	+++++	++++	+++	Yes, +
RGS4	1q21–22	+++	+++	+++	Yes, ++
GRM3	7q21–22	+++	+	++++	No, ++
DISC1	1q42	+++	++	++	Not known
G72	13q32–34	+++	++	++	Not known
DAAO	12q24	++	+	++++	Not known
PP3CC	8p21	+	++++	++++	Yes, +
CHRNA7	15q13–14	+	++	+++	Yes, +++
PRODH2	22q11	+	++++	++	No, +
Akt1	14q22–32	+	+	++	Yes, ++

The ratings are of course subjective and transient.

eliminate 3p as a candidate region. The findings for chromosome 6p generated considerable excitement.[135] It was thought at first that the susceptibility locus on 6p accounted for up to 30% of the variance in the families studied,[133] but it is now considered that only about 10% of the variance may be accounted for by this region. Another problem is that rather a large region of chromosome 6 was implicated by the positive studies, perhaps a segment containing hundreds of genes. It will be no easy task to narrow the search further.[135]

A study using a different approach – linkage to individual traits rather than to diagnosis – also implicates chromosome 6p. Arolt et al.[136] tested for linkage between poor eye-tracking (a phenotypic marker associated with schizophrenia) and markers on chromosome 6p in eight multiply affected families. The positive evidence for linkage was quite strong, but requires replication. Another large, international collaboration[137] was established to test positive reports of linkage

Fig. 32 Schizophrenia susceptibility genes and the strength of evidence in four domains. Reproduced from Harrison PJ, Weinberger DR. *Molec Psychiat* 2005;**10**: 40–68[129] with permission from Nature Publishing Group.

Fig. 33 Linkage studies aim to show association between parts of chromosomes and characteristics or diseases so as to indicate the area of a chromosome that appears conserved or transmitted with that disease

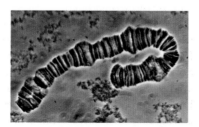

between schizophrenia and an area of the long arm of chromosome 22 – D22S278. These authors concluded that if a susceptibility gene exists in this area, then its contribution to the overall liability to schizophrenia is rather small, perhaps some 1%. Recent functional genomic studies have taken this further (see below).

Association studies

Association studies examine the association of disease and markers in individuals from different families.[127] For example, we could say that a population association exists between a gene and schizophrenia if those with schizophrenia were more likely than suitable controls to have a specific version of the gene.[138] A major disadvantage of association studies is that the DNA marker must be tightly linked to the disease gene. This is in contrast with the linkage method, which can detect linkage over relatively large distances.

To date, the most consistently replicated finding in this area is an allelic association between HLA-A9 and paranoid schizophrenia, which has been found in seven out of nine studies.[115,139] This association could account for about 1% of the liability to the disorder. A negative association has recently been found between schizophrenia and HLA-DR4,[140] lending support for immunological explanations for the aetiology of schizophrenia.

Anticipation

Anticipation is an inheritance pattern within a pedigree whereby disease severity increases and age of onset decreases in successive generations. This phenomenon has been described in several neuropsychiatric disorders, including fragile X, Huntington's disease and some spinocerebellar degenerations.[141] These diseases represent a new class of disorders caused by unstable DNA sequences that can change in each generation. Such mutations depart from Mendelian inheritance, and have a highly variable phenotype with wide-ranging age at onset, both of which are well-known characteristics of schizophrenia. Anticipation has been reported in families affected with schizophrenia in two or more generations,[142,143] and some specific trinucleotide repeats have been demonstrated in some samples.[144,145]

The future for molecular genetic epidemiology

Linkage studies using non-parametric approaches in nuclear families and association studies using functional polymorphisms are taking over from the standard parametric lod score approach in the study of the genetics of schizophrenia.[115] As more susceptibility genes for schizophrenia are discovered there will be a move towards investigation of larger samples that are capable of detecting genes of smaller and smaller effect. Rapid and inexpensive methods of genotyping and sequencing using microchip technology are being developed and will lead to further increases in efficiency.

The exemplar of the new, molecular genetic paradigm comes from studies of the catechol-O-methyltransferase (COMT) gene, undertaken largely by Weinberger and colleagues.[146] COMT is an enzyme that catalyses the breakdown of catecholamine neurotransmitters, including dopamine, in the brain. The COMT gene on 22q11 contains a functional polymorphism (Val[108/158]Met) affecting the enzyme's activity; the Met allele produces a four-fold decrease in activity,[147] leading to increased availability of dopamine in the prefrontal cortex.[148] Dopaminergic dysfunction in frontal brain regions is fundamental to schizophrenia,[149] where cognitive dysfunction is prominent. The Val allele confers an increased risk for schizophrenia,[150] but is extremely common in the general population.[151] In healthy adults, the COMT genotype affects cognitive performance; studies find better executive function in people with the Met/Met genotype.[146,152] Egan et al. showed that performance on the Wisconsin card sorting test, a frontal executive test of strategy and set shifting, was dependent upon the COMT alleles present, that performance was, as expected, worse in people with schizophrenia and, with the same allelic-dependent response, intermediate between schizophrenia and controls in first-degree relatives. The results are summarized in Fig. 34.

Thus, we are now in a position where we have some target genes with biologically plausible effects that may contribute to liability to schizophrenia, or to a relevant endo-phenotype[153] that is the true risk

Fig. 34 Performance on the Wisconsin card sorting test is dependent on the COMT alleles present. As expected, people with schizophrenia performed worse on this test; the performance of first-degree relatives was intermediate between schizophrenia patients and controls, with the same allelic-dependent response. Reproduced from Egan MF, et al. *Proc Natl Acad Sci USA* 2001;**98**(12): 6917–22.[146] © 2001, National Academy of Sciences, USA.

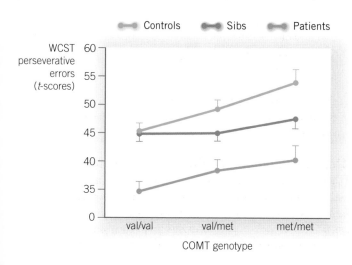

Fig. 35
Ventricle:brain ratio in normal subjects and subjects with schizophrenia. This breakthrough study led people to believe all cases might be different from all controls, but this has proved not to be the case. Reproduced from Johnstone EC, et al. *Lancet* 1976;**2**: 924–6[154] with permission from Elsevier.

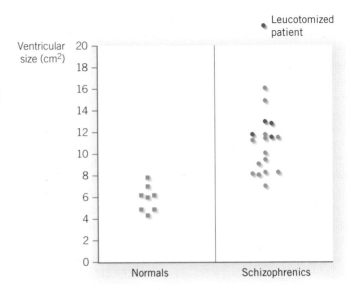

Fig. 36 MRI coronal views from two sets of monozygotic twins discordant for schizophrenia showing subtle enlargement of the lateral ventricles in the affected twins (b, d) as compared with the unaffected twins (a, c), even when the affected twin had small ventricles.
Reproduced with permission from Suddath RL, et al. *New Engl J Med* 1990;**322**:789–94.[156] Copyright © 2002 Massachusetts Medical Society. All rights reserved.

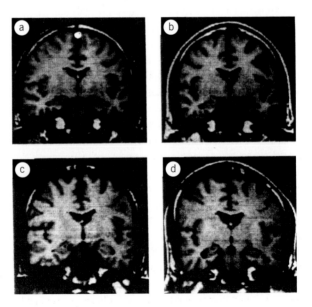

modifier for the disorder. It is likely that, just as for other complex disorders such as heart disease, liability for disease is built up in layers, with genes contributing additively or multiplicatively, and interacting with environmental factors such as hypoxic stress, emotional stress or street drugs – multiple genes of small effect, rather than any single major gene that is necessary or sufficient.

The argument thus far has concentrated on a psychological or cognitive endo-phenotype, but there must be a structural correlate. Neuroimaging studies indicate small group differences between people with schizophrenia and those without (Fig. 35), first identified in terms of cerebral ventricle enlargement by Johnstone et al.[154] 30 years ago; their study helped put biological research in schizophrenia back on the agenda.

We don't really know if these abnormalities in cerebral structure that may underpin cognitive mechanisms of psychosis are genetic or environmental, or more likely a combination.[155] The magnetic resonance imaging (MRI) study by Suddath et al.[156] of monozygotic twins discordant for schizophrenia shows that the presence of genetic risk does not account for all variance in structural differences associated with schizophrenia, and that environmental or gene–environment interactive risks are involved (Fig. 36).

The most consistent finding is that schizophrenia patients have larger lateral ventricles than controls, with many small imaging studies yielding almost as many potential findings. A recent meta-analysis of MRI data by Wright et al.[157] has identified areas of consistency, and allowed the field to focus on specific areas and think about which systems may be involved (Fig. 37).

Structural brain abnormalities such as these are relatively large scale as explanations for the psychological abnormalities in schizophrenia and their explanations in terms of aberrant connectivity.[158,159] The true structural endo-phenotype, which may itself rely on an abnormality at a more detailed, molecular level, is likely to be operating at the level of neurons, glia, their connections and interactions. Harrison and Weinberger[160] have produced a speculative review of the neuropathology and genetics of schizophrenia, the relationship between them, and their functional convergence. Imaging studies suggest that the subtle morphological correlates of schizophrenia outlined above sit beside localized alterations in the morphology and molecular composition of specific neuronal, synaptic and glial populations in the hippocampus, dorsolateral prefrontal cortex and dorsal thalamus. These findings suggest a view of schizophrenia not only as a disorder of connectivity, but also of the synapse.

Recent identification of several putative susceptibility genes in addition to COMT, such as neuregulin, dysbindin, DISC1, RGS4, GRM3 and G72, provide a way to flesh out the rather vague notions of multiple genes of small effect being involved. Having said that, a putative causal allele that would explain predisposition to schizophrenia has been identified only for COMT. Harrison and Weinberger speculate that the genes may all converge functionally upon schizophrenia risk via

Fig. 37 Meta-analysis of structural MRI studies of schizophrenia 1988–99.

Reproduced with permission from Wright IC, et al. *Am J Psychiat* 2000;**157**(1):16–25.[167] © 2000, American Psychiatric Association.

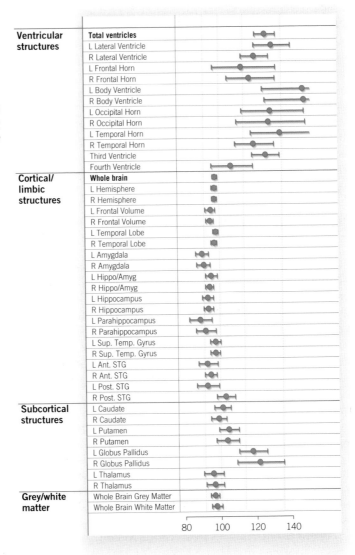

Ventricular structures	Total ventricles	
	L Lateral Ventricle	
	R Lateral Ventricle	
	L Frontal Horn	
	R Frontal Horn	
	L Body Ventricle	
	R Body Ventricle	
	L Occipital Horn	
	R Occipital Horn	
	L Temporal Horn	
	R Temporal Horn	
	Third Ventricle	
	Fourth Ventricle	
Cortical/ limbic structures	Whole brain	
	L Hemisphere	
	R Hemisphere	
	L Frontal Volume	
	R Frontal Volume	
	L Temporal Lobe	
	R Temporal Lobe	
	L Amygdala	
	R Amygdala	
	L Hippo/Amyg	
	R Hippo/Amyg	
	L Hippocampus	
	R Hippocampus	
	L Parahippocampus	
	R Parahippocampus	
	L Sup. Temp. Gyrus	
	R Sup. Temp. Gyrus	
	L Ant. STG	
	R Ant. STG	
	L Post. STG	
	R Post. STG	
Subcortical structures	L Caudate	
	R Caudate	
	L Putamen	
	R Putamen	
	L Globus Pallidus	
	R Globus Pallidus	
	L Thalamus	
	R Thalamus	
Grey/white matter	Whole Brain Grey Matter	
	Whole Brain White Matter	

an influence upon synaptic plasticity and the development and stabilization of cortical microcircuitry. Glutamate transmission mediated by NMDA may be especially implicated, though there are also direct and indirect links to dopamine and GABA. Hence, there is a correspondence between the putative roles of the genes at the molecular and synaptic levels and the existing understanding of the disorder at the neural systems level. The authors suggest that characterization of a core molecular pathway and a "genetic cytoarchitecture" would be a profound advance in understanding schizophrenia, and may have equally significant therapeutic implications.

Functional genomics and proteomics

Technological advances in molecular biology as opposed to genetics now allow the analysis of gene expression in terms of either the amount of mRNA expressed or of proteins synthesized. These get progressively closer to the biological substrate of the purpose of genes – coding for proteins that then undergo post-translational changes and take part in biological processes. Thus, we may begin to further explore the "genetic cytoarchitecture" suggested by Harrison and Weinberger. Techniques to examine mRNA and protein expression are conceptually different from molecular genetics, as well as technically distinct, because they treat genes as dynamic properties of tissues (whatever is examined), rather than fixed effects of individuals. To undertake gene expression analysis, one needs a sample of the relevant tissue, in this case the brain, so these analyses are presently undertaken on postmortem tissue. There are prospects for analysis on peripheral tissue or cell culture. Thus, the techniques represent a new amalgam and extension of genetics, neuropathology and imaging.

Several studies have now been published, with interest aroused concerning reproducible up-regulation of several members of the apolipoprotein L family located in a high-susceptibility locus for schizophrenia on chromosome 22 (Fig. 38) in an area implicated by the more traditional genetic studies reviewed above.[161] Such findings are "causally agnostic" in that the causes of this up-regulation may be primarily genetic, environmental or due to a combination, and are not the subject of investigation. The findings may be relevant to pathophysiology though, acting through phospholipids as vital components of normal cell membranes, or as antioxidants protecting against stress triggered by infection, hypoxia or other mechanisms. Replication will confirm these techniques as crucial new tools for schizophrenia research.

Fig. 38 Contemporary gene expression analysis in schizophrenia.
Changes in regulation may themselves be primarily genetic or as a result of environmental interactions. Adapted from Mimmack ML, et al. *Proc Natl Acad Sci USA* 2002;**99**(7): 4680–5.[161] © 2002, National Academy of Sciences, USA.

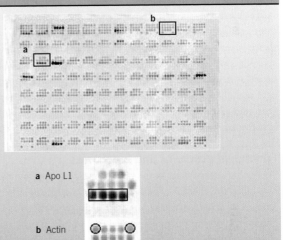

Schizophrenia

a Apo L1

b Actin

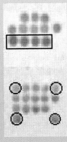

Control

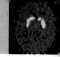

Environmental risk factors

Simple additive models suggest that at least 20–30% of the variance in liability to schizophrenia may be attributable to non-genetic factors. The environment can no longer be considered a "nuisance variable" by psychiatric geneticists, just as it should not be by clinicians who acknowledge the sometimes intimate relationship between their patients' experiences, their mental state and quality of life. Epidemiological clues, such as the city risk factor, serve as indicators of true risk modifiers or causes, and triggers, such as life events, are well known. What makes people vulnerable? As we identify putative genes for schizophrenia, so too must we identify the factors in the environment with which they may interact.

Many environmental risk factors appear to operate before, around or soon after birth (Fig. 39). Alone, or together with the effects of genes, they may underpin or be manifestations of neurodevelopmental aspects of the disorder[23] that have been outlined above.

> *Additive models suggest that at least 20–30% of the variance in liability to schizophrenia may be attributable to non-genetic factors*

Category of risk factor	Specific risk	Best estimate of effect in terms of n-fold effect
Genetic	MZ twin of someone with schizophrenia	46
	DZ twin of someone with schizophrenia	14
	Child or sibling	10
	Parent	5
Childhood developmental	Childhood CNS infection	5
	Delayed milestones	3
	Speech and language problems	3
Pre- and perinatal environment	Perinatal brain damage	7
	Rhesus incompatibility	3
	Unwanted pregnancy	2
	Severe under-nutrition (first trimester)	2
	Maternal influenza (second trimester)	2
	Season of birth (winter/spring)	1.1

Fig. 39 "Best estimate" effect sizes of various genetic and environmental risk factors for schizophrenia (expressed as odds ratios or relative risks)

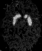
"People with schizophrenia, as a group, experience a greater number of labour and delivery complications than controls"

"However, labour and delivery complications, but not necessarily significant hypoxia, are relatively common in the population and are only rarely associated with schizophrenia. Other factors must play a part in a causal constellation"

Pregnancy and birth complications

People with schizophrenia, as a group, experience a greater number of labour and delivery complications than controls.[162,163] Inspection of the particular complications associated with schizophrenia suggests that foetal hypoxia and the biological cascade that ensues from hypoxic stress may be the common mechanism underlying these associations.[164–166]

However, labour and delivery complications, but not necessarily significant hypoxia, are relatively common in the population and are only rarely associated with schizophrenia. Other factors must play a part in a causal constellation. Taking a static approach, a particular neuronal system must be damaged or extra vulnerability such as genetic predisposition must be required for schizophrenia to arise. A more dynamic, developmental view might include chance as a factor, which, along with other specific factors, determines a self-perpetuating trajectory towards psychosis,[50] as already mentioned.

Complications of pregnancy have also been associated with schizophrenia, of which the most robust are: prenatal exposure to influenza,[167–169] prenatal nutritional deprivation,[170,171] low maternal weight,[32] rhesus incompatibility[99] and prenatal stress.[172,173] The effect sizes associated with these prenatal risk factors are usually small (between 2 and 3), indicating that they are unlikely to be single causal agents. The association with influenza may reflect an effect related to maternal immunological responses to infection, as mentioned earlier. The association with rhesus incompatibility may be mediated through foetal hypoxia resulting from haemolysis.

Perinatal and early childhood brain damage

Findings from a 28-year follow-up of a Finnish birth cohort have shown that children with perinatal brain damage (defined as neonatal convulsions, low Apgar scores, asphyxia, intraventricular haemorrhage or abnormal neurological signs in the newborn period) were some seven times more likely to develop schizophrenia in adulthood than the remainder of the cohort.[37] Data from the same Finnish cohort showed that individuals who had suffered a viral CNS infection during childhood were almost five times more likely to develop schizophrenia than the comparison group.[174] The relative incidence of schizophrenia was particularly high among a group of 16 individuals who had contracted neonatal Coxackie B meningitis during an epidemic in one maternity unit. The relative effects of CNS infection are rather higher than those found for influenza in ecological studies,[123,168] possibly due to reduction in measurement error and misclassification of viral exposure. In this study, patients with schizophrenia were also more likely to have a history of childhood epilepsy.

This area of investigation has been taken forward over recent years through a remarkable set of investigations exploiting maternal and cord blood samples that were saved on a number of birth cohorts in North America collected routinely within private medical insurance schemes. There was direct evidence of an association with prenatal infection in that maternal cytokine levels were elevated in a dose–response manner in the mothers of offspring who later developed schizophrenia.[175] Furthermore, the offspring of mothers with elevated levels of total IgG and IgM and antibodies to herpes simplex virus type 2 were at increased risk for the development of schizophrenia and other psychotic illnesses in adulthood.[176]

Foetal maldevelopment

Several studies have shown that people with schizophrenia are more likely to have had low birth weight and decreased head circumference at birth.[177] Minor physical abnormalities and dermatoglyphic abnormalities, which are thought to represent "fossilized" evidence of early developmental deviance, occur to excess in schizophrenia, as do cytoarchitectural changes, which are consistent with disturbances of development during gestation.[177] These indicators of foetal maldevelopment may be due to a genetic process[114] or may indicate environmental insult to the foetus. A study of MZ twins discordant for schizophrenia has shown that the affected co-twin had more markers of prenatal developmental disruption than the unaffected twin.[178,179]

Season of birth

There is a small increase in risk for schizophrenia [odds ratios (OR) of around 1.15] among individuals born in winter to early spring.[180] The reason for this "season of birth" effect is unknown,[181] although it may be a crude proxy for exposure to viral or other environmental events such as infection.

Heavy cannabis intake

Some drugs, such as amphetamine, have long been known to precipitate a paranoid psychosis that can closely resemble schizophrenia during intoxication. Indeed, this fact, combined with amphetamine's effects on dopamine, is part of the evidence underpinning the dopamine hypothesis of schizophrenia described in the sections on treatment. Other drugs are also implicated.

Cannabis, too, can cause a psychotic state during intoxication, but the question as to whether it can trigger an ongoing schizophrenia syndrome, thereafter, remains unresolved; the pendulum is swinging towards this possibility just as the legislative frameworks governing its

"Some drugs, such as amphetamine, have long been known to precipitate a paranoid psychosis that can closely resemble schizophrenia during intoxication"

"The question as to whether it can trigger an ongoing schizophrenia syndrome, thereafter, remains unresolved; the pendulum is swinging towards this possibility just as the legislative frameworks are becoming more liberal"

Study	Study design (n), Year of enrolment	Gender	Number of participants	Follow-up (years)	Age of cannabis users (years)	Outcome, n (%)	Diagnostic criteria/ instrument
Swedish conscript cohort Andreasson et al.[182]	Conscript cohort (~50,000) 1969–70	Male	45,570	15	18	In-patient admission for schizophrenia, 246 (0.5)	ICD-8
Zammit et al.[185]	Conscript cohort (~50,000) 1969–70	Male	50,053	27	18	Hospital admission for schizophrenia, 362 (0.7)	ICD-8/9
NEMESIS van Os et al.[186]	Population-based (7076) 1996	Male and female	4104	3	18–64	(a) Any levels of psychotic symptoms, 33 (0.9) (b) Pathology level of psychotic symptoms, 10 (0.3) (c) Need for care, 7 (0.2)	BPRS
Christchurch study Fergusson et al.[184]	Birth cohort (1265) 1977	Male and female	1011	–	21	Psychotic symptoms, NA	SCL-90
Dunedin study Arsenault et al.[183]	Birth cohort (1037) 1972–3	Male and female	759	11	15–18	Schizophreniform disorder: (a) Symptoms (b) Diagnosis, 25 (3.3)	DSM-IV
Overall risk†							

BPRS, Brief Psychiatric Rating Scale; NEMESIS, Netherlands Mental Health Survey and Incidence Study; SCL-90, 90-item Symptom Check List.

†Beta of multiple linear regression.

Fig. 40 Summary of epidemiological studies on cannabis use and schizophrenia.
Reproduced from Arseneault et al. *Br J Psychiatr* 2004;**184**: 110–7[187] with permission from the Royal College of Psychiatrists.

use are becoming more liberal in some countries. Heavy cannabis consumption at the age of 18 was associated with an increased risk of later psychosis (OR 2.3) in a large cohort of military conscripts in Sweden.[182] A dose–response relationship was convincing. However, despite recent and important cohort studies, two from New Zealand,[183,184] the reanalysis of the Swedish data[185] and a study from the Netherlands,[186] the direction of causality remains uncertain and is probably complex. The results are summarized in Fig. 40, taken from Arsenault et al.[187]

Early and heavy use are probably to be avoided or should be a target for intervention either at the public health or clinical level.

Definition of cannabis use	Risk of schizophrenia-related outcome given cannabis use OR (95% CI)	Adjusted risk OR (95% CI)	Confounding variables controlled for	Dose–response relationship	Specificity of risk factor	Specificity of outcome
Used cannabis >50 times at age 18 years	6.0 (4.0–8.9)	**2.3 (1.0–5.3)**	Psychiatric diagnosis at conscription Parents divorced	Yes	No	NA
Used cannabis >50 times at age 18 years	6.7 (4.5–10.0)	**3.1 (1.7–5.5)**	Diagnosis at conscription IQ score Social integration	Yes	Yes	NA
Cannabis use at baseline (age 16–17 years)	3.25 (1.5–7.2)	**2.76 (1.2–6.5)**	Disturbed behaviour and cigarette smoking Place of upbringing	Yes	Yes	NA
	28.54 (7.3–110.9)	24.17 (5.44–107.5)	Age Gender Ethnic group			
	16.15 (3.6–72.5)	12.01 (2.4–64.3)	Single marital status			
DSM-IV cannabis dependent at age 21 years	2.3 (2.8–5.0)	**1.8 (1.2–2.6)**	Education Urban dwelling Discrimination Time-varying covariates	NA	Yes	NA
Users by the age of 15 years and continued at 18 years	β = 6.91 (5.1–8.7)* 4.50 (1.1–18.2)	β = 6.56 (4.8–8.34) **3.12 (0.7–13.3)**	(e.g. nicotine, alcohol, other drug dependence) Fixed covariates (e.g. gender, IQ, parental criminality) Social class Psychotic symptoms prior	NA	Yes	Yes
		2.34 (1.69–2.95)	to cannabis use			

†The adjusted odds ratios included in the calculation of the overall risk for psychosis are in bold type. Results across studies were homogeneous (test for heterogeneity: $Q = 2839$ on four degrees of freedom; $P = 0.585$).

However, whether there is some shared liability to both schizophrenia and to such use remains a possibility, as does an additive effect of cannabis on top of that underlying vulnerability. There is evidence of an interaction between a functional polymorphism in the serotonin transporter gene and the cognitive and emotional effects of ecstasy.[188] There are preliminary reports of a similar interaction between COMT and cannabis. If cannabis (Fig. 41) can cause schizophrenia de novo and on its own, then the apparent increase in consumption in the general population over recent decades, perhaps with increases in its strength, should have led to corresponding increased rates of psychosis. As noted above, the question of trend over time is complex but is consistent with that notion.

It is, however, certain that use and abuse of "street" drugs (Fig. 42) is common in people with schizophrenia, and complicates management enormously. Clinical services should have very close ties with drug and alcohol services. Neither should we forget smoking tobacco, which is again very common and contributes to the excess mortality in this group.

Fig. 41 The cannabis plant. Picture courtesy of Royal Botanic Gardens, Kew, UK.

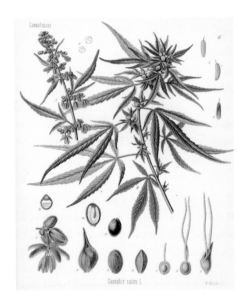

Fig. 42 Cannabis use is common in people with schizophrenia, just as in people without it. Cannabis can certainly complicate treatment of schizophrenia, although initial use may ameliorate the psychological symptoms.

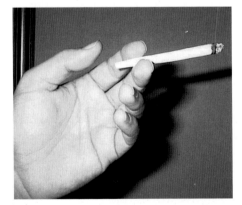

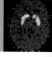

PREVENTION

Despite substantial scientific advances over the past 15 years, the diagnosis of schizophrenia remains one of clinical judgement and the aetiological precursors for any individual patient are most often unknown. Therefore, intervening to reduce the risk of developing schizophrenia on an individual patient basis is a mammoth task.[189] Alternatively, health systems can undertake broader public health initiatives to reduce the incidence of schizophrenia.[190,191] Improved antenatal and obstetrical care is one good example. However, there is no compelling evidence for a reduction in the incidence of schizophrenia in countries that have improved their obstetrical services over the past 20 years.[192] That does not discount an effect of improved obstetrical care, but if such an effect has occurred its contribution to the risk of developing schizophrenia is at best small. Similar prevention efforts include the reduction and better treatment of head injuries. Again, the effect of head injuries is small.

Much research has provided clear evidence that many patients show (in retrospect) a lifelong pattern of subtle neurological and cognitive deficits that presage the emergence of the typical symptoms (most commonly) during adolescence or early adulthood.[38,190] Many patients may have delayed motor milestones, neurological deficits, lower IQ than expected, attentional and related cognitive difficulties, and impairments of social and scholastic achievement. These findings, however, are non-specific and do not of themselves lead to any earlier clinical detection of schizophrenia.

Several other researchers have attempted a related strategy of trying to intervene just before the onset of overt psychosis, at a time when the patient is exhibiting prodromal signs of illness but has not yet decompensated fully into psychosis.[192,193] This approach, at least a little more focused than (earlier) intervention based on childhood biobehavioural precursors, is important because it offers the (intuitive) prospect that early intervention may prevent disease deterioration and resultant disabilities. There is now evidence from studies in patients who are in the prodromal stage of illness that treatment with an atypical antipsychotic medication can delay the onset of psychosis in these at-risk groups.[192–194] Whether this approach can actually ultimately prevent schizophrenia occurring or whether such early intervention could make the course of the illness more benign is as yet unknown. Since exposing people who do not have a diagnosis of schizophrenia to medications carries with it risks and serious ethical concerns, until the results of more research come in it is not (yet) justifiable to take such an aggressive approach to medication interventions.[195] Nevertheless, this is a major area of interest with promise for the future.

> *Despite substantial scientific advances over the past 15 years, the diagnosis of schizophrenia remains one of clinical judgement*

> *Intervening to reduce the risk of developing schizophrenia on an individual patient basis is a mammoth task*

> *Since exposing people who do not have a diagnosis of schizophrenia to medications carries with it risks and serious ethical concerns, until the results of more research come in it is not (yet) justifiable to take such an aggressive approach to medication interventions*

55

Putative approaches for preventative and early intervention models of schizophrenia management are illustrated in Figs 43 and 44.

Genetics
- identify "at-risk" genes
- genetic counselling

Eliminate risk factors

Obstetric complications
- improve antenatal care
- decrease labour complications
- improve neonatal care

reduces

Vulnerability to develop schizophrenia

Pre-morbid neurobehavioural manifestations

Symptoms of schizophrenia

Fig. 43 Prevention of schizophrenia

Fig. 44 Early intervention for schizophrenia

Stages	Possible intervention strategies
Pre-morbid neurobehavioural antecedents	Unknown
Prodromal stage	• Antipsychotic medications • Cognitive behavioural therapy • Psychosocial support
First episode of psychosis	• Antipsychotic medications • Cognitive behavioural therapy • Psychosocial support

SOME HISTORY OF THE CLINICAL CONCEPT AND OTHER THOUGHTS ABOUT SCHIZOPHRENIA

"As a "functional" psychosis, the syndrome is often defined as being without cause. This is ridiculous"

As a "functional" psychosis, the syndrome is often defined as being without cause, or at least one thought of as acting on the brain rather than the psyche.[196] Known *sufficient* causes of the syndrome, such as some drugs and epilepsies, lead to a diagnosis being excluded in contemporary classifications, including the two used here, and in the most recent major classifications used for research – namely, DSM-IV[8] and ICD-10.[9] This is ridiculous.

The harmful effect that this persistence of a Cartesian split between mind and body may have had on the search for the causes of schizophrenia is well recognized.[3,197] It rests uneasily with contemporary, neurobiological formulations of the mechanisms of normal and abnormal mental phenomena. We won't explore reductionist arguments,[198] but any good explanation of any psychological event cannot be thought of as complete unless brain function (or dysfunction) is included. A theory of schizophrenia has to explain everything about the disorder if it is to be complete. However, an incomplete explanation can still be a useful one, one explaining delusions or difficulties in social functioning, for instance.

Some features of the schizophrenia syndrome can be recognized in classical Greek literature.[199] The Ancients considered them to be separate from the agitations or manic states that were accompanied by fever, conditions that they called the "phrenitides". This is similar to the distinction, mentioned above, that some still make today between functional and organic psychosis, something that may be holding back our understanding (see below). At a clinical level, it was during the 19th century that nosologists and physicians began to group together these syndromes not associated with known organic states (such as general paralysis of the insane or neurosyphilis) into distinct mental disorders.

Dementia praecox

Kraepelin (Fig. 45) is widely credited with the first description of what would today be recognized as schizophrenia,[200] as well as having developed a number of modern clinical psychiatric practices and an experimental approach to understanding psychology. Kraepelin used the term "dementia praecox" to cover the syndromes of catatonia, hebephrenia and dementia paranoids, including them all into a single entity within the functional, "endogenous" psychoses. Kraepelin distinguished this group from manic depression, and from the dementia associated with old age, which he later named Alzheimer's disease in recognition of the

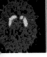
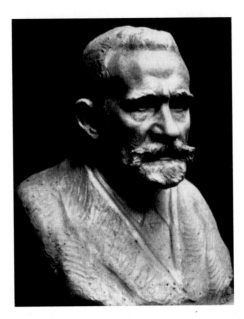

Fig. 45 Emil Kraepelin 1856–1926, an enormously influential German psychiatrist, himself influenced by the experimental psychology of Wilhelm Wundt. A concise biography of Kraepelin can be found at http://www.uni-leipzig.de/~psy /eng/kraep-e.html. Photo courtesy of the Royal College of Psychiatrists.

contribution to its characterization by his friend and colleague. Depression and melancholia were already considered as separate. Kraepelin's first description of dementia praecox was published in 1896 in the fifth edition of his textbook, *Psychiatrie*,[20] refined 3 years later in the sixth edition. This is usually read in the eighth edition,[201] when he had included in the definition the "dementia simplex" described by Pick[202] and by Diem.[203] It is well worth reading, still seeming fresh and obviously composed on the basis of detailed clinical observation and considerable thought.

The term *dementia praecox* used in this way did not arise out of the blue; it was based on other descriptions of the 19th century. Pinel[204] had used "demence" to describe psychotic states, and Morel[205,206] used the term "demence precoce" when he reported psychosis beginning in the teenage years. Snell[207] had already separated primary paranoid states (*primare Verrucktheit*) from mania and melancholia, Kahlbaum[208] had distinguished catatonia, and Hecker[209] had described the phenomenology of hebephrenia, a description upon which Kraepelin drew later in his first, 1896, account. These authors tended to view these states as separate entities until Fink[210] described mixed states of catatonia and hebephrenia. Kraepelin further described the phenomenology and clinical characteristics of dementia praecox, but stressed the young age at onset and deteriorating course as the major distinguishing features of dementia praecox. He was one of the first clinicians to really include the long view in classification.

Schizophrenia

Twelve years after Kraepelin's first account, Eugene Bleuler (Fig. 46) questioned the importance of youth and deterioration when he outlined his views of the prognosis of dementia praecox.[21] He felt that the *splitting* or *tearing apart* of the psychic functions that occurred in the disorder was a more unifying characteristic than either age at onset or deteriorating course (although he acknowledged the view that the syndrome did usually deteriorate). Having written with touching deference in his text to Kraepelin's contribution, he went on to use the term "*Schizophreniegruppe*", the group of schizophrenias, to describe this. The first part of this term has stuck and is best described in a later account.[22]

Bleuler stressed the phenomena of a disintegration of personality, with disturbances of formulation and expression of thinking. Perception and the sense of reality were altered, and there was an incongruous effect. He considered that these were common to a group of heterogeneous psychotic conditions that could occur in clear consciousness without obvious brain disease. In the 1911 account, Bleuler had also divided these phenomena into the *primary* or fundamental psychological dysfunctions of altered associations (disordered thought form and structure), altered affect, ambivalence and autism, and the *secondary* features such as delusions and hallucinations that he considered to be the result of, or secondary to, the primary features.

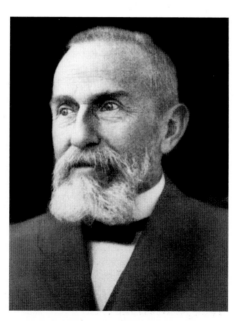

Fig. 46 Eugene Bleuler, Swiss psychiatrist and psychologist. Born 30 April 1857, Zollikon near Zürich, died 15 July 1939, Zollikon. Photo courtesy of the Royal College of Psychiatrists.

Bleuler intended to narrow the concept of schizophrenia by emphasizing these underlying or primary features; he considered delusions and hallucinations as non-specific. The opposite happened, possibly due to the emerging zeitgeist of psychoanalysis.[211] Bleuler's primary disturbances were difficult to define specifically and were seen widely by psychiatrists in their patients' states of mind. Attention is drawn to them here because they infer the notion that several systems of the mind and brain are disturbed in schizophrenia, and that such disturbances may exist independently of the more dramatic phenomena that are stressed in descriptions of the clinical syndrome, e.g. hallucinations. Minkowski[212] summarized the views of others[213] and incorporated his own into a view of schizophrenia (although he still called it dementia praecox) as a disorder of the harmonious interplay between several mental functions. This view is regaining popularity, particularly as explained by a mechanism of disordered neural connectivity (see below). It underlies the approach taken here to examine the thesis in terms of risk factors reflecting, and possibly affecting, several psychological and brain systems, both at the time of psychosis and before it begins.

The schizophrenia concept continued to develop over subsequent decades, yielding rather than culminating in the current, operational, clinical definitions. The concept is more fluid in many areas of research (discussed by Castle and Murray[214]), concentrating on individual symptoms rather than the syndrome. The modern definitions owe a lot to the phenomenological school, particularly regarding positive psychotic phenomena.

Kurt Schneider was central to steering definitions towards an exclusively phenomenological one when he published a list of the symptoms that he considered to be of first-rank importance (Fig. 47), or most useful when trying to make a diagnosis of schizophrenia.[215] He

Fig. 47 Symptoms that Schneider considered of first-rank importance in making a diagnosis

Hearing your thoughts spoken aloud
Hearing voices talking about you – third person hallucinations
Hearing a voice(s) describing what you're doing (running commentary)
Somatic hallucinations
Thought withdrawal and/or insertion
Thought broadcasting
Delusional perception
Feelings or actions made, controlled or influenced by forces outside the self

considered other symptoms as less discriminatory, or of second-rank importance.

With the addition of criteria for altered social functioning and chronicity, and exclusion criteria such as predominating depression and organic brain conditions, these first-rank symptoms form the basis of the modern operational definitions, though none is necessary or specific. Schneider himself was rather modest in describing his list, suggesting that it might help the diagnosis of schizophrenia, not shape the concept for decades to come.

These modern operational classifications (so-called diagnostic menus) followed the demonstration in the early 1970s of unacceptable discrepancies in definitions of schizophrenia used by English and American psychiatrists.[216] This work precipitated the development and widespread use of operational diagnostic criteria, now available across the spectrum of psychiatric conditions. The trap of mistaking reliability for validity in these definitions is well recognized,[1] but they have made much research evidence at least reliable, or more comparable between studies.

All operational systems rely on a largely cross-sectional definition of schizophrenia as a clinical syndrome. The core features are certain types of auditory hallucinations, particularly voices heard talking in the third person, changes in thought construction and form and, finally, bizarre delusions which often involve a person's ego boundary, such that thoughts may be available to others or a person is influenced by outside forces. These positive, psychotic phenomena, comprising the core diagnostic features, are heavily influenced by Schneider's ideas. They usually occur together with changes in an individual's behaviour or social functioning. There may also be so-called negative features, such as restriction of the range of emotions and decreased ability to initiate thoughts and ideas; these are Kraepelin's and Bleuler's legacy, recently developed further by Andreasen.[1] Some criteria, such as the early DSM, incorporate items regarding short-term course, something which may have a major impact on research into outcomes, and even on aetiological research, where predisposing and precipitating factors may be confused with those that perpetuate the disorder.[92]

None of the core features of schizophrenia is pathognomonic, although the presence of at least one, in the absence of an obvious organic precipitant, such as drug intoxication, is essential for the diagnosis. As Bleuler proposed, several psychological systems can be affected, including perceptions in various modalities, the generation, construction and inferential use of thoughts, emotions and volition.

Andreasen[1] has summarized her own and others' views of schizophrenia as it approached its centenary. She emphasized the polythetic nature of schizophrenia and the division of its features into positive and negative, along the lines suggested originally by Jackson[217] and later by Crow.[218] Andreasen notes that the array of signs and symptoms classified as positive or negative is often summarized according to the range of cognitive and emotional domains involved. Overall, schizophrenia must involve many brain systems or sub-systems (Fig. 48).

There are two competing explanations in anatomical terms. On the assumption that the functions and systems in Fig. 10 can each be localized to specific brain regions, the first suggests that schizophrenia may be a condition such as multiple sclerosis or cerebral lupus, where multiple, discrete lesions in different sites produce a varied and heterogeneous condition.[219,220] The second, again reminiscent of Bleuler, Stransky and Minkowski, draws upon ideas of distributed parallel processing.[68,219] Abnormalities of the connectivity or "wiring" of the brain may produce multiple effects depending upon the circuits involved and the site of the problem. The complexity of brain circuitry would ensure a multiplicity of inter-related symptoms[221,222] and other cognitive effects manifest only with specific tests.

Since the early 1970s, this latter idea of disordered functional connectivity in schizophrenia has been amenable to direct investigation by

Fig. 48 Relationship between features of schizophrenia and neural systems

Symptom	Neural system or sub-system
Positive	
Hallucinations	Perception
Delusions	Inferential thinking
Disorganized speech/thought form	Language
Disorganized/bizarre behaviour/catatonia	Behavioural monitoring and secondary to other psychotic phenomena
Negative	
Alogia	Conceptual fluency
Affective blunting	Emotional expression
Anhedonia	Experiencing pleasure
Avolition	Volition
Other	
Motor signs at onset	Extrapyramidal and other motor systems
Cognitive deficits	Wide range of cortical and sub-cortical systems

The diagnosis of affective psychosis versus schizophrenia rests largely on the single affective item that can have a range of expression other than blunting in other disorders, and in schizophrenia as well. The multiplicity of systems affected suggests to many an underlying difference in integrative or connectivity mechanisms.

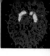

functional neuroimaging techniques, first[223] by crude single-photon emission tomography (SPET), and now by high-resolution SPET, positron emission tomography (PET) and functional magnetic resonance imaging (fMRI). Cognitive tasks, such as verbal fluency, are used to activate and suppress activity in specific cortical areas, and normal subjects are compared with those with schizophrenia in terms of space and time.[224] As originally suggested by Wernike,[225] a disturbance of connections between the prefrontal and temporal cortices would fit many clinical data concerning schizophrenia, and frontostriatal and frontocerebellar circuits are also posited as important. Recent ideas concerning causation might also fit in with such a connectivity model, including the timing of possible aetiological events in mid-pregnancy,[226–228] when relevant connections are being formed.[229] These ideas are considered again in the section on causes.

McGuire and Frith[230] noted that the direct evidence for dysconnectivity in schizophrenia is as yet largely circumstantial, "its popularity owing as much to conceptual appeal as it does to scientific data". However, there is an opportunity to test, in biological terms, the model put forward by Bleuler. The field is reviewed by Friston.[231]

These ideas ignore many other attempts, particularly in continental Europe (see Hirsch and Shepherd[232] for a review), to identify and define the clinical borders of schizophrenia within mental illness. The review here has stressed the widespread nature of the psychopathology in the clinical syndrome even when this is defined narrowly by modern criteria. The syndrome is a cross-sectional one, but may be better thought of in longitudinal terms, with the clinical syndrome and its subsequent course as part of its evolution;[227] this influences modern practices in terms of diagnosis and underpins the contemporary early intervention movement.

In terms of the brain and mind, what we call schizophrenia could alternatively be regarded as the effects of schizophrenia, not a disease in itself. If so, then the true definition of schizophrenia remains almost as elusive as it has been over the rest of the century, but at least we know where to look, in the structure and functioning of the brain, as well as the phenomena it generates.

> **In terms of the brain and mind, what we call schizophrenia could alternatively be regarded as the effects of schizophrenia, not a disease in itself**

Problems with categorical definitions and operational criteria

One fundamental problem concerns causes, or rather the lack of them, in our definitions. Medicine likes to classify disease on the basis of cause and mechanism. We should not be too hard on psychiatry for not adopting this stance because we are unsure of the true causes and mechanisms for many psychiatric disorders, except for those where this

> **One fundamental problem concerns causes, or rather the lack of them, in our definitions**

forms part of the definition, such as post-traumatic stress disorder. Here, building a cause into the definition means that we assume the category is distinct from other anxiety disorders, and we can't be certain of that either. We do a strange thing with schizophrenia in that whenever we have a possible organic cause for the syndrome, like epilepsy, we say this isn't schizophrenia. We've become paralysed by the old idea of schizophrenia as a functional psychosis and rule out the diagnosis when there is gross neuropathology or brain disease. This is despite the accumulating evidence (and common sense view) that there is an underlying neurobiological substrate for the production of these features.

Another problem concerns the boundaries, not between different psychotic syndromes, although these overlap, coexist or evolve in interesting ways, but between normality and psychosis. Psychologists have long been interested in personality dimensions in psychosis, such as schizotypy, that may share some genetic causes with schizophrenia, and in cognitive vulnerability. Recent psychiatric and epidemiological interest has quickened, particularly due to the work of van Os and Verdoux, who have shown not only that responses similar to individual psychotic symptoms (not the syndrome) are relatively common in young adults, but that they may share some of the same risk factors and, perhaps, causes. Similar findings have come from both the Epidemiological Catchment Area programme[71] (ECA) and from the National Comorbidity Survey in the USA. Endorsement of probes for psychotic symptoms is common in these general population surveys. Data from the latter are represented in Fig. 49.[233]

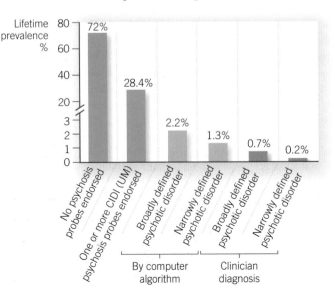

Fig. 49 Lifetime prevalence of endorsement of probes for psychosis in the US population, and lifetime prevalence of broadly and narrowly defined psychotic disorder according to computer algorithm and expert clinicians. Drawn from data in Kendler KS et al. *Arch Gen Psychiat* 1996;**53**: 1022–31.[233]

TREATMENT

At present, there is no cure for schizophrenia, although, as already noted (Fig. 9) there are a range of outcomes.[234,235] Treatments are most effective when they are used in combination: pharmacotherapy, psychotherapy, family and social support. It is crucial that patients, family members – and also clinicians – appreciate that while we now have a range of drug treatments for schizophrenia, it is not as simple as one drug being "better" than another. Each has different indications. For example, clozapine is the drug of choice for severe schizophrenia. Each of the typical antipsychotics and the atypicals risperidone, olanzapine, quetiapine, ziprasidone and aripiprazole (but not clozapine) are appropriate choices for early ("first-episode") schizophrenia and also for other stages of the illness.

Family involvement and support are also crucial components for success. Increasingly, as outcome improves, the need to ensure the provision of adequate vocational, housing and allied community resources will be more apparent.

The components of comprehensive disease management for schizophrenia are highlighted in Fig. 50.

Outcome of treatment has been variously defined and can be measured along many dimensions (see Fig. 51). Lehman has operationalized these outcomes into proximal and distal outcomes (see Fig. 52).

The evolution of various pharmacological therapies for schizophrenia has given rise to several pharmacological models for the neuroreceptor targets of antipsychotics and the influence of various neuroreceptors on specific symptoms and side effects. Primary among the pharmacological models, and still dominant after decades of research, is the dopamine hypothesis – a model that focuses on imbalances in dopaminergic activity.

"Treatments are most effective when they are used in combination: pharmacotherapy, psychotherapy, family and social support"

Medication treatment
Individual supportive therapy
Cognitive and psychosocial therapies
Family psychoeducation and support
Social support
Case management
Housing
Financial support
Vocational support

Fig. 50
Comprehensive care for schizophrenia

Fig. 51 Multidimensional outcomes in schizophrenia.

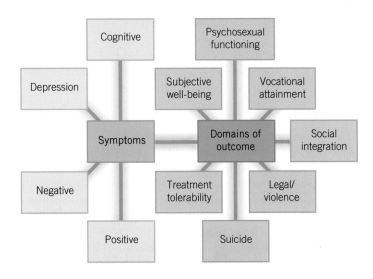

Fig. 52 Proximal and distal outcomes in schizophrenia.
Reprinted with permission from Lehman AF. Developing an outcomes-oriented approach for the treatment of schizophrenia. *J Clin Psychiatry* 1999;**60**: 30–5.[234] © 1999, Physicians Postgraduate Press.

Proximal	Distal
Positive symptoms	Functional status
Negative symptoms	Quality of life
Disorganization	Family well-being
Relational functions	Public safety
Side-effects	
Ancillary symptoms	

According to the dopamine hypothesis of schizophrenia, hyperactivity of the mesolimbic dopaminergic pathway mediates symptoms of psychosis, while hypoactive dopaminergic pathways mediate negative and cognitive symptoms. Although antipsychotics that inhibit dopamine transmission reduce the activity of hyperactive dopaminergic pathways, they also trigger side effects, such as EPS, and increased prolactin secretion, by diminishing levels of dopamine in pathways where dopamine excess was not initially a problem.

In addition to dopamine, other neurotransmitters that have been associated with schizophrenia include serotonin, GABA (gamma-aminobutyric acid), glutamate, norepinephrine, acetylcholine, and various neuropeptides (Fig. 53). The relative influence and importance of these non-dopamine neurotransmitters remains to be fully defined. However, as research into the neurophysiology of schizophrenia progresses, it is becoming apparent that manifestations of the illness may actually represent the sum of multiple neurochemical abnormalities.

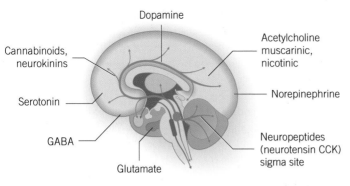

Fig. 53 Potential sites of antipsychotic drug action

Figure 54 reflects an updated, more current, form of the dopamine (DA) hypothesis. It illustrates how dopamine receptor abnormalities in both the cortical and subcortical areas of the brain are postulated to result in the positive and negative symptoms of schizophrenia. On the bottom right of this figure (A), a pathway for the induction of positive symptoms is shown. This illustrates the dopamine hypothesis in its earliest, 'classic', form. Briefly, it postulates that in the subcortex, an *excess* of dopamine together with *hyperstimulation* of D_2 dopamine receptors, is associated with the appearance of positive symptoms of schizophrenia.

On the left (B), an expansion of the dopamine hypothesis that was first proposed in the early 1990s is shown. It postulates that a *deficit* in dopamine, together with *hypostimulation* of dopamine receptors in the prefrontal cortex (PFC), results in the negative symptoms and cognitive

Fig. 54 Differential regional impact of dopamine dysfunction in schizophrenia

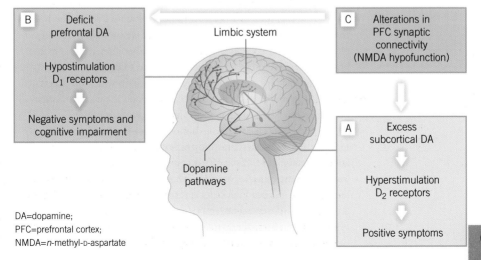

DA=dopamine;
PFC=prefrontal cortex;
NMDA=*n*-methyl-D-aspartate

67

impairment seen in schizophrenia. This theory was based on clinical observations that cognitive impairment was linked to abnormalities in the prefrontal cortex and that, in animal models, induced dopamine depletion in the prefrontal cortex resulted in cognitive deficits.

The top portion of Fig. 54 (C) illustrates the newest expansion of the dopamine hypothesis. This new addition proposes that both types of dopamine abnormalities – the coexisting subcortical dopamine excess and the prefrontal dopamine deficit – derive from an alteration in synaptic connectivity in the prefrontal cortex, and that this alteration is associated with N-methyl-D-aspartate (NMDA) hypofunction.

"Typical" and "atypical" antipsychotics – what's in a name?

Typical and atypical antipsychotic medications form the backbone of disease management for schizophrenia.[235,236] The decision to choose a typical antipsychotic or an atypical antipsychotic medication – and which drug to use within either class – is complex. The decision should be made by the patient in collaboration with his/her doctor. Response to previous medications, sensitivity to side-effects and the pattern of the illness in that patient are all important considerations. It makes very good sense to involve family members in this decision, particularly since they may be the best judges as to how well the patient responded to previous drug treatments. It is also helpful to review any available literature to compare and contrast each drug, so that the patient is informed as to which drug might be best for his/her circumstances. At the present time, the evidence for selecting one atypical over another is incomplete and there is a need for more comparative studies between these agents. Additionally, we are learning more now about the adverse effect profile of the atypical antipsychotics. Therefore, it is likely that practice patterns and the information accrued to determine such changes will evolve further and at a rapid pace over the next 5 years. With this in mind, it is important to understand the current distinctions between typical and atypical antipsychotic medications.

At the outset, the reader is cautioned that the current nomenclature to classify and describe antipsychotic medications is controversial and confusing.[237,238] Older ("first generation", "conventional", "typical") antipsychotics are drugs that possess antipsychotic efficacy but are also associated with extrapyramidal side-effects (EPS). This is an essential difference between typical and atypical medications.[238] However, even here, there is a considerable "grey area" with this distinction because (i) some drugs classified as typical antipsychotics

	Typical	Atypical
Extrapyramidal side-effects	+++	+/−
Hyperprolactinaemia	+++	+/−
Binding to mesolimbic D_2 dopamine receptors	+++	++
Efficacy for negative symptoms	+	++
Efficacy for cognitive symptoms	−	+
Effect on broader domains of outcome (e.g. depression, suicide)	+/−	+

Fig. 55 Proposed features that differentiate atypical from typical antipsychotic medications

(e.g. loxapine) may (particularly when given in low dose) have a low propensity to induce EPS, and (ii) some of the atypicals (e.g. risperidone) can induce EPS, particularly if used in moderate to high doses. Also, neither typicals nor atypicals constitute a homogeneous group and there is wide intragroup variability (especially in adverse effect profile) between agents. Therefore, the notion that the term "atypical" appropriately describes a well-aggregated group of drugs of similar mechanism, efficacy or side-effect profile is inherently misleading. It is, however, the best working hypothesis for the present time. Other aspects which are proposed to distinguish typical from atypical antipsychotics are highlighted in Fig. 55.

❝Neither typicals nor atypicals constitute a homogeneous group and there is wide intragroup variability (especially in adverse effect profile) between agents❞

Typical antipsychotics

The first antipsychotic medication, chlorpromazine, when originally used in anaesthesia, was noted to diminish hallucinations and delusions, and to have a calmative effect.[239] Because of these effects, antipsychotic medications were originally termed "major tranquillizers". The various classes (or subcategories) of drugs and examples of commonly used drugs are highlighted in Fig. 56.

Mechanism of action

Although it is unclear how these drugs work, the proposed mechanism of action of both typical and atypical antipsychotics is that they block dopamine (D_2) receptors.[240,241] An exception to this is ariprazole, which acts as a partial agonist at D_2 receptors. The actual scientific evidence in support of this claim comes from various sources and is summarized in Fig. 57. This is also illustrated in Fig. 58.

Fig. 56 Classes of antipsychotic medications

Class	Example
Typical	
Butyrophenone	Haloperidol
Phenothiazine	
Aliphatic	Chlorpromazine
Piperidine	Thioridazine
Piperazine	Trifluoperazine
Thioxanthene	Fluphenthixol
Diphenylbutylpiperidine	Pimozide
Substituted benzamide	Sulpiride
Atypical	
Dibenzodiazepine	Clozapine
Benzisoxazole	Risperidone
Thienobenzodiazepine	Olanzapine
Dibenzothiazepine	Quetiapine
Benzisothiazolyl	Ziprasidone
Dihydrocarbostyril	Aripiprazole
Phenylindol	Sertindole
Dibenzothiepine	Zotepine

Fig. 57 Evidence for blockade of dopamine receptors as a mechanism of action of antipsychotic medications

Amphetamine, which promotes dopamine (DA) release, induces a schizophrenia-like psychosis
Antipsychotics (typicals) block DA D_2 receptors to an extent that correlates with their clinical potency
Cis-fluphenthixol isomer (which blocks D_2 receptors), but not *trans*-fluphenthixol (inert isomer), is an effective antipsychotic
Response to treatment with typical antipsychotics has been shown to correlate with changes in plasma homovanillic acid, the metabolite of dopamine
Recent PET studies confirm the need for typical antipsychotics to achieve above 60% D_2 receptor occupancy to be clinically effective

These drugs also cause EPS as a direct result of the basal ganglia.[238,241] Imaging studies of the binding of drugs to D_2 receptors, as assessed using PET, indicate that there is a very narrow dosing range or "window" within which one can achieve antipsychotic efficacy with typicals without causing EPS (Figs 12, 58 and 59).[242–245] Doses below this D_2 binding threshold (approximately 60% D_2 receptor occupancy) are clinically ineffective for treating schizophrenia. Doses that increase the D_2 occupancy to 70% or above will induce EPS. The atypicals, in general, have a wider therapeutic window (see later).

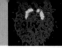

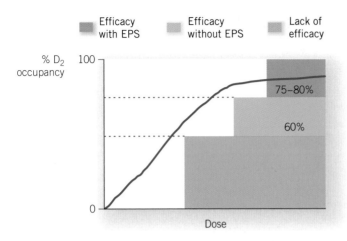

Fig. 58 Dopamine receptor occupancy and clinical outcomes

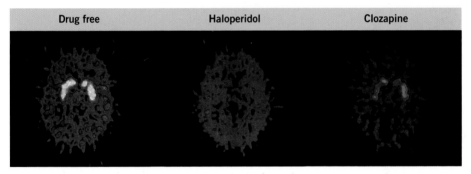

Fig. 59 Neuroimaging of antipsychotic action shows strong dopamine D₂ binding with haloperidol but weak D₂ binding with clozapine

Clinical efficacy

Typical antipsychotics are effective, with an acute onset of antianxiety effect followed by a reduction in positive symptoms.[235,246] Compared with placebo relapse rates of upwards of 80%, these drugs also reduce relapses over the course of the illness.[247] However, this advantage is lost if the dose is too low.[235] Long-acting intramuscular formulations are available and are effective options, especially when poor compliance is a concern.[248]

Unfortunately, many patients respond very poorly to these drugs.[249] Additionally, typical antipsychotics are of limited effect, and can even worsen negative symptoms and depressive symptoms in patients with schizophrenia. They also have no appreciable effect on cognitive deficits and may even aggravate these.[250,251]

Type	Mechanism	Risk factors	Treatment
Acute dystonia Oculogyric crisis and torticollis	Acute hypodopaminergia in basal ganglia	Young males, high dose, high potency, typical antipsychotics	Immediate – oral or IM anticholinergic Subsequent – reduce dose or change to atypical antipsychotic or add oral anticholinergic
Parkinsonism Bradykinesia Tremor Cog-wheel rigidity	Basal ganglia D_2 blockade	Dose related, more with typical antipsychotics	Reduce dose or add oral anticholinergic Switch to an atypical antipsychotic
Akathisia Motor and subjective restlessness	Basal ganglia D_2 blockade Low iron also relevant?	Low serum iron Dose related, more with typical antipsychotics	Reduce dose or add benzodiazepine/beta-blocker Switch to atypical antipsychotics

Fig. 60
Extrapyramidal side-effects of antipsychotic medications

Adverse effects

Common neurological side-effects from typical antipsychotic medications are acute dystonia, akathisia and Parkinsonism.[238,252] These effects and their management are highlighted in Fig. 60. The addition of an anticholinergic drug, reduction of the dose of the typical antipsychotic or switching to an atypical antipsychotic (now the preferred option) are the management choices.

Tardive dyskinesia (a more long-term effect) occurs at a rate of 5% per year for the first 5 years of treatment, with rates up to 50% in elderly populations (see Fig. 61).[253,254] There is evidence that clozapine reduces

Fig. 61 Tardive dyskinesia

Description	Antipsychotic-induced abnormal involuntary movements (facial, truncal, limbs)
Risk factors	Age Female gender Organic brain disease Prominence of negative symptoms Typical antipsychotic medications (predominantly) • high dose • long duration of treatment
Management	Change antipsychotic – atypical is preferred choice, clozapine has indication for treatment of tardive dyskinesia Other (less preferred choices) include adjunctive treatment with vitamin E or amantidine

Definition	Idiosyncratic patient reaction to (predominantly) typical antipsychotic medications, characterized by: • muscle rigidity • altered consciousness • pyrexia • autonomic instability • elevated creatinine phosphokinase
Risk factors	• organic brain disease • pre-existing dehydration • pre-existing agitation • rapid titration and intramuscular use of typical antipsychotic medications
Management	• stop antipsychotics • hospitalize • supportive measures – hydration, correct any electrolyte imbalance • dantrolene and/or bromocryptine may reduce morbidity of NMS episode • if another antipsychotic required, then use an atypical antipsychotic: start 2 weeks after resolution of NMS

Fig. 62 Neuroleptic malignant syndrome

tardive dyskinesia and there is less but emergent data for the other agents. There is evidence now that the atypicals are approximately 10 times less likely to induce tardive dyskinesia.[255]

Less than 0.5% of patients exposed to treatment with typical (much less with atypicals) antipsychotics may develop neuroleptic malignant syndrome (NMS) (Fig. 62).[256,257]

Non-neurological side-effects of typical antipsychotics are high-lighted in Fig. 63.[258]

Current indications for the use of typical antipsychotics

In America, typical antipsychotics are infrequently used. In Europe, the pattern is less clear and the change in prescribing pattern from typicals to atypicals is inconsistent across countries. The reasons for this are varied and include economic reasons as well as a more widespread belief in Europe in the continued benefit of treatment with typicals.

Pharmacoeconomic studies indicate that atypical antipsychotics are more economical than the typicals, despite their disproportionately higher prescription costs[259,260] (because of the rapid evolution of this literature and its specificity to each country, only an overview/recent articles are provided here and the topic is not covered in detail in this

Fig. 63 Non-neurological side-effects of typical antipsychotic medications

Type	Treatment
Orthostatic hypotension	Lower doses, hydrate; change to an atypical antipsychotic if persistent
Hyperprolactinaemia • Amenorrhoea • Galactorrhoea • Complex neuro-endocrine/metabolic effects	Change to prolactin-sparing atypical antipsychotic
Sexual dysfunction • Decreased libido • Impotence • Ejaculation failure • Anorgasmia	Evaluate carefully; consider change to atypical antipsychotic
Sedation	Use less medication or less sedating antipsychotic
Anticholinergic effects • Blurred vision • Dry mouth • Constipation	Change to atypical antipsychotic
Cardiac arrhythmias • Benign • Torsade de pointes, fatal/sudden death	Increased risk with thioridazine, risk with other antipsychotics considered low
Weight gain	More common effect with atypical antipsychotics; molidone may be the least weight-inducing typical antipsychotic

text). It appears, but is not conclusively proven by the available literature, that the atypicals are cost-effective due to less hospitalizations.

The proposed superior efficacy and enhanced tolerability of atypicals and the extent to which such attributes should dictate whether the atypicals replace the typical agents is a contentious issue in European psychiatry. A systematic overview and meta-regression analyses of 52 randomized controlled clinical trials of atypical agents – amisulpiride, clozapine, risperidone, olanzapine, quetiapine and sertindole – reported that the evidence for superior efficacy of atypicals over typicals was weak and inconsistent between the atypicals.[261] In addition, the authors reported that when the haloperidol dose was below/equal to 12 mg/day, atypicals proved only comparable to typical antipsychotics in efficacy and drop-out, although the new drugs still had less EPS. The authors concluded that there was insufficient evidence to support atypical antipsychotics being more effective or better tolerated than typical antipsychotics; specifically, the authors went on to recommend: "Conventional antipsychotics should be used in the initial treatment of an episode of schizophrenia unless the patient has previously not responded to these drugs or has unacceptable extrapyramidal side-effects". There is also another study which compared olanzapine and haloperidol over 1 year of treatment.[262] The authors found a comparable response between olanzapine and haloperidol, with less EPS but more weight gain on olanzapine. Another meta-analysis of randomized controlled clinical trials of atypical agents found that clozapine, amisulpiride, risperidone and olanzapine were overall more efficacious than typicals; the remaining atypicals were equiefficacious with the typical antipsychotics.[263] They also noted that the dose of haloperidol did not affect the results. They concluded that some atypicals are substantially more efficacious than typical antipsychotics, while others are not. Also, the comparison between atypical and typical antipsychotic medications – and between atypicals – has now become more complex over time because of the emergent side-effect profile of atypicals. However, the debate over which medication is the right choice will continue. Consumers advocate a wider availability and greater access to all medications – both typical and atypical antipsychotics. At the time of writing, typical antipsychotics are being prescribed less and less in the USA (the pattern in Europe is less clear), but they are still used in patients who are responding well and without EPS. Typicals are also used (liquid, tablet and short-acting intramuscular forms) for acute agitation.[246] However, there are now available several short-acting injectable atypicals and also a long-acting injectable atypical antipsychotic. Recent authoritative guidelines now support the preferential use of atypical anitpsychotic medications for the treatment of schizophrenia.[264–267]

> *"Typical antipsychotics are being prescribed less and less ... Recent authoritative guidelines now support the preferential use of atypical antipsychotics ... However, the debate over which medication is the right choice will continue"*

Atypical antipsychotic medications
Mechanism of action

Clozapine is the prototypic atypical antipsychotic medication and, in contrast to typical medications, it binds to many neurotransmitter receptors.[268] It also binds less than typical agents to dopamine D_2 receptors, even though it is more efficacious than typical antipsychotics. The pharmacology differs substantially between these drugs and it is at present unclear whether such differences reflect different mechanisms of action. It is also unclear whether these account for any reported differences in efficacy, adverse effect profiles, or both, between the currently available atypical antipsychotic medications.

The adverse effect profile of atypical antipsychotics is covered in detail in the section on management. The relative receptor binding profiles for each of these agents is given in Figs 64 and 65.

Fig. 64 Scheme of receptor antagonistic binding profile of antipsychotic medications

Scheme of receptor antagonistic binding profile of antipsychotic medications					
Drug	**D_2**	**$5\text{-}HT_{2A}$**	**H_1**	**α_1**	**ACh**
Haloperidol	+++	–	–/+	+	–/+
Thioridazine	+	+	+	++	+·+
Trifluoperazine	++	–	–/+	+/–	+·+
Amisulpride	+	–	–	–	–
Clozapine	+/–	++	+++	+	+·+
Risperidone	+	+++	–	+	–
Olanzapine	+	++	++	+	+·+
Quetiapine	+/–	+/–	–	++	–
Sertindole	+	+	–	+	–
Aripiprazole	*	++	–	–	–
Ziprasidone	+	+++	–	++	–
Zotepine +	+	–	+	–	

D_2 = dopamine D_2 receptor; $5\text{-}HT_{2A}$ = 5-hydroxytryptamine receptor, type 2A; H_1 = histamine H_1 receptor; α_1 = alpha 1 adrenoceptor; ACh = acetylcholine receptor; – = no significant receptor binding antagonism; +/– or –/+ = minimal receptor antagonism; + = receptor antagonism; ++ = moderate antagonism; +++ = strong antagonism. * high affinity binding at D_2 but functions as partial agonist

Fig. 65 Safety and tolerability of antipsychotics

Antipsychotics safety and tolerability							
Item	**Typ**	**Clz**	**Ris**	**Olz**	**Qtp**	**Apz**	**Zip**
EPS	+-+++	±	±-+++[a]	±-+[a]	±	±-+	±-+[a]
TD	+++	±	±-+	±(?)	±(?)	±(?)	±(?)
Somnolence	±-+++	+++	±	+	++	±	±
Prolactin	+++	±	+++	±	±	±	±
Weight	±-++	+++	+	+++	+	±	±
Dyslipidaemia	±-+	+++	+	+++	++	±	±
DM	±-+	+++	+	+++	++	±	±
QT_c	±-+++	++	+	+	+	±	++
Orthostatic BP↓	±-+++	+++	++	+	++	±	±

[a] = dose-related; ± = none to minimal; + = mild; ++ = moderate; +++ = marked compared to placebo rate

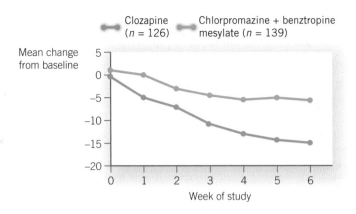

Fig. 66 Clozapine versus chlorpromazine: BPRS score in treatment-resistant patients. Reproduced with permission from Kane J, et al. The Clozapine Collaborative Group. *Arch Gen Psychiat* 1988;**45:** 789–96.[269] Copyright © 1988, American Medical Association. All rights reserved.

Clozapine

Clozapine was introduced in 1990 in the USA and has subsequently gained wide use in the USA and Europe, on the basis of the compelling findings of a carefully conducted study comparing clozapine and chlorpromazine in patients with severe ("treatment-refractory") schizophrenia.[269] At the end of the 6-week trial, 30% of clozapine-treated patients were classified as treatment responders compared with 4% of the chlorpromazine-treated group (Fig. 66). Subsequent studies and experience in clinical practice affirm clozapine's position as the treatment of choice for patients with treatment-refractory schizophrenia.[270–272] Clozapine is also indicated where patients are unable to tolerate an adequate dose of antipsychotic because of side-effects. This indication for "neuroleptic intolerance" focuses specifically on extrapyramidal side-effects and tardive dyskinesia. Clozapine has extremely low levels of EPS and, on current evidence, does not appear to cause tardive dyskinesia. In fact, clozapine is now the treatment of choice for patients with tardive dyskinesia.[273]

An important development for clozapine therapy, and for other atypical antipsychotic medications, is the understanding of its differential effects on various symptom and behavioural domains (see Figs 51, 52 and 67). Although the effect may lie predominantly in clozapine's low propensity to induce EPS, there is substantial evidence that negative symptoms of schizophrenia can be ameliorated, at least in part, with clozapine therapy.[274] There is also evidence that clozapine may possess thymoleptic properties and thus be beneficial in treating co-morbid mood disturbance in schizophrenia. Related to this are some important findings suggesting that clozapine might reduce suicidality in patients with schizophrenia,[275] including those from the InterSePt study, a multi-centre randomized controlled trial.[276] This trial is con-

"Thirty per cent of clozapine-treated patients were classified as treatment responders compared with 4% of the chlorpromazine-treated group ... Studies and experience in clinical practice affirm clozapine's position as the treatment of choice in treatment-refractory schizophrenia "

Fig. 67 Use of clozapine and other atypical antipsychotic medications for specific patient subgroups

Schizophrenia
- co-morbid substance abuse
- co-morbid aggression
- tardive dyskinesia

Schizophrenia refractory to antipsychotic trials with typical (and other atypical) antipsychotics

sidered further on page 109. There are also data to suggest that clozapine is effective in reducing persistent aggression in patients with schizophrenia.[277] Although less well studied to date, there is accruing information that clozapine may also be of particular benefit in patients with co-morbid substance abuse.[278] Finally, there is considerable evidence that clozapine can produce modest improvements in cognitive functioning in patients with schizophrenia.[250,251] This may be a particularly important effect because of the detrimental impact of cognitive dysfunction on overall level of functioning and on the capacity for vocational rehabilitation.[279]

Clozapine is typically initiated at 25 mg per day and increased by 25 or 50 mg per day over the first 10 days of treatment. Therapeutic doses of 300–600 mg are required. It may be necessary in maintenance therapy to titrate up to the maximum dose of 900 mg in order to obtain an adequate response. A trial of clozapine of 4–6 months duration is indicated in patients who are poor responders to other treatments.[280] Most patients respond within the first month of therapy, but some may show a delayed response in the third or fourth months of therapy. It is thought that the determination of the plasma level of clozapine may be helpful to maximize efficacy.[280] Plasma levels above 400 ng/ml are recommended.

The main reason for the restricted and low use of clozapine is its side-effect profile. The side-effect profile and that of the other atypical antipsychotics is given in Fig. 68. The major side-effect particularly associated with clozapine therapy is agranulocytosis.[281] This effect is seen in approximately 0.38% of patients receiving clozapine and typically occurs (80% of cases) within the first 18 weeks of therapy. This is the reason why weekly blood work is performed for the first 6 months of therapy and alternate weeks thereafter in the USA. The frequency of testing in the UK is weekly for the first 6 months and then monthly; the testing frequency differs between countries. Risk factors for agranulocytosis are older age and female gender. The concomitant use of drugs known to cause agranulocystosis should be avoided – consequently, carbamazepine is contraindicated with clozapine therapy. The careful monitoring of white cell counts as well as the rapid and effective use of granulocyte-stimulating factor when agranulocytosis develops

Type	Mechanism	Risk factors	Treatment
Neurological	See Fig. 59; uncommon with atypical antipsychotics		
Seizures	Clozapine lowers seizure threshold	Rapid dose escalation; dose dependent – 6% at 600 mg/day	Reduce dose; add anticonvulsant
Non-neurological	See Fig. 60; in general, these are less common with atypical antipsychotics		
Weight gain	Complex, possibly related to antagonism at serotonin histamine and other receptors	Higher baseline Body Mass Index	Dietary advice and restriction, exercise; change to an alternative antipsychotic; antiobesity agents
Diabetes mellitus	Unknown, possibly related to antagonism of serotonin receptors	Obesity; family history of diabetes mellitus	Switch to another antipsychotic medication; routine diabetic care

Fig. 68 Side-effect profile of atypical antipsychotic medications

have led to a negligible mortality rate with this event. Once a patient develops agranulocytosis, they must never again receive clozapine.

Seizures, generalized and myoclonic, are another serious side-effect of clozapine. Seizures occur in approximately 3–6% of patients and are dose dependent. They can be managed by reducing the dose (and going slow in titrating dose increases) and/or adding an anticonvulsant (valproic acid being the most frequent choice). A seizure is not an indication to discontinue clozapine. There have also been reports of clozapine-induced myocarditis and pulmonary embolism.[282,283] These are certainly infrequent. In contrast, weight gain and metabolic disturbances are common in clozapine-treated patients.[284] On current evidence, clozapine is most likely among all the atypical antipsychotics to cause weight gain and to cause metabolic disturbances.[285–289] Most patients gain some weight but a substantial proportion (variously estimated; conservatively 50%) of patients will become obese while on clozapine (obesity is currently defined as a Body Mass Index of 29 or greater). This may be a reason for the patient to stop taking clozapine and it is certainly a concern for the patient and the clinician regarding the long-term consequences of neuroleptic-induced weight gain. Allied to this, patients may have elevated cholesterol, plasma lipid levels, glucose intolerance (approximately 10% of patients) and diabetes mellitus.[290,291] Uncommonly, but nevertheless of great concern, some patients experience diabetic ketoacidosis. These effects are serious and a reason why clinicians now tend to favour the use of other atypical antipsychotics over clozapine.

The main reason for the restricted and low use of clozapine is its side-effect profile

Risperidone

Unlike clozapine, risperidone has a more targeted profile of neuro-transmitter binding, with particular predeliction for dopamine and serotonin receptors.[268] Risperidone is widely used in all phases of psychosis (i.e. first episode, maintenance, treatment refractory).[292] Risperidone is best prescribed at low doses (1–4 mg/day) for the treatment of schizophrenia. Some patients may require doses of 6 mg and above, but in such instances the patient is likely to experience EPS and sometimes also sedation. Like clozapine, risperidone is effective in treating positive symptoms of schizophrenia.[293] It is also partially effective in treating negative symptoms.[294] Risperidone may reduce co-morbid mood symptoms in patients with schizophrenia and is now (like many of the atypical antipsychotics) also a treatment choice for patients with bipolar disorder.[295] Risperidone has also been shown in several studies to modestly improve cognitive function in patients with schizophrenia.[250,296] There is evidence that this improvement may be most pronounced in verbal memory. There are no substantive data yet published to suggest that risperidone reduces suicidality. However, it has been shown to reduce persistent aggression in patients with schizophrenia.[297] Importantly, this drug is also available in liquid form and there are strong data now pointing to superior efficacy and tolerability of risperidone over haloperidol in the acute management of agitated psychotic patients.[246,298] Risperidone is also available in a wafer ("melt-in-your-mouth") degradable tablet format, which may enhance medication compliance.

Risperidone is also available in a long-acting injectable (depot) form.[299] The availability of a long-acting form of an atypical antipsychotic (risperidone microspheres; others are under development) represents a substantial advantage for the maintenance care of patients with schizophrenia, particularly for those patients with poor medication compliance. Information to date shows that risperidone microspheres act as an effective antipsychotic, with an adverse effect profile similar to the oral forms of risperidone.[299,300] The medication is dispensed by injection at a usual dose of 25–37.5 mg every 2 weeks. Because it takes time for the drug to build up in the bloodstream, the patient must also be on an oral antipsychotic for the first 2 weeks after starting risperidone microspheres. There are ongoing longitudinal and observational studies to evaluate the long-term effectiveness of the new treatment approach.

Oral risperidone is used at lower doses of 1–2 mg in patients with a first episode of psychosis. Emsley reported equiefficacy (65% response rate) between risperidone and haloperidol in first-episode patients.[301] There is also evidence that risperidone is more effective than

"Risperidone is best prescribed at low doses (1–4 mg/day), although occasionally some patients may require doses of 6 mg and above"

"Risperidone microspheres represent a substantial advantage for maintenance care, particularly for patients with poor medication compliance"

haloperidol in the maintenance treatment of schizophrenia. In a 1-year trial, there was a 23% relapse rate in patients receiving risperidone compared with a 35% relapse rate in the haloperidol-treated group.[302] There is also evidence to suggest that risperidone is effective for a proportion (perhaps 11–30%) of patients with treatment-refractory schizophrenia.

Risperidone has a favourable side-effect profile. It has a low propensity to cause extrapyramidal side-effects, although this is dose dependent and will occur in many patients receiving doses at or above 6 mg/day. Based on current knowledge, it has a substantially lower risk of tardive dyskinesia than with typical antipsychotic medications. In a 1-year trial, incidence of tardive dyskinesia was 0.6%.[302] Risperidone is associated with weight gain and diabetes, but considerably less so than most other atypical antipsychotics, particularly clozapine. In one comparison, using a British general medical database, of risperidone with olanzapine and with typical antipsychotics, risperidone was associated with less diabetes and with less lipid abnormalities.[303] Risperidone-treated patients only gained 5 lb during a 1-year trial.

Olanzapine

Olanzapine is another atypical antipsychotic of proven efficacy.[292] It possesses a pleomorphic receptor binding pattern to neurotransmitters, with marked affinity for serotonergic and muscarinic receptors.[268] Typical doses of olanzapine for the acute and maintenance treatment of patients with schizophrenia are between 10 and 20 mg daily. The current approved upper limit for treatment is 20 mg/day, although it is not uncommon for experienced clinicians to prescribe doses above 20 mg/day for patients with treatment-refractory schizophrenia.[304] Olanzapine is available in oral tablet and rapidly disintegrating tablet forms, as well as in an acute intramuscular formulation.

Olanzapine has a broadly similar efficacy profile to clozapine and risperidone, in that it is effective in treating positive, negative, depressive and cognitive symptoms of schizophrenia.[305] The effects on negative symptoms are comparable to those seen with the other agents.[306] Olanzapine is effective for co-morbid mood symptoms and in fact has an approved indication in the USA for the treatment of bipolar disorder. In the pivotal registration trial, olanzapine was superior to haloperidol in ameliorating co-morbid depressive symptoms, with 57% of this effect being attributable to a direct effect on depression.[307] There are several studies which indicate that cognitive performance is enhanced with olanzapine therapy.[250,308]

In a recent 1-year comparative study, olanzapine proved superior to both haloperidol and risperidone on several measures of cognitive function.[308] There is at present little evidence that olanzapine reduces

> **The current approved upper limit for olanzapine is 20 mg/day, although it is not uncommon to prescribe doses above 20 mg/day for treatment-refractory schizophrenia**

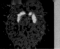
suicidality in patients with schizophrenia. There is strong evidence that olanzapine in a short-acting, injectable preparation is an effective and well-tolerated treatment for the acutely agitated psychotic patient.[309] There is also some early evidence that olanzapine may be an effective treatment in patients with co-morbid substance abuse.[310]

Olanzapine is an effective antipsychotic for use in first-episode schizophrenia, with typical doses being 5–10 mg. In a 6-week study, which examined efficacy in first-episode patients, 67% of olanzapine-treated patients responded compared with 29% of haloperidol-treated patients.[311] In another initial report of a study of 2 years duration, olanzapine was superior to haloperidol in first-episode patients.[312] Olanzapine is also frequently prescribed as a maintenance treatment. In a study of 1 year of treatment, 14% of olanzapine-treated patients relapsed compared with 19% of haloperidol-treated patients.[313] Another 1-year study of olanzapine versus haloperidol showed comparable outcomes overall, although cognitive performance was better in patients receiving olanzapine.[262]

Olanzapine is effective in treating refractory schizophrenia.[314] An early trial of olanzapine in refractory patients proved beneficial for 7% of the olanzapine-treated group.[315] Olanzapine was also reported to perform well compared with clozapine in a large European trial.[316] Another trial comparing olanzapine (up to 30 mg per day) with risperidone, haloperidol or clozapine found that olanzapine was comparable to clozapine in this patient population.[317]

Olanzapine has a favourable side-effect profile with respect to its low propensity to induce EPS or tardive dyskinesia, but this is now overshadowed by its weight and metabolic adverse effect profile. Extrapyramidal side-effects are not common and while there is a relationship between emergence of EPS and increasing dose of olanzapine, this relationship is much weaker than is observed with risperidone. Olanzapine has a low rate of tardive dyskinesia. In an analysis of treatment-emergent tardive dyskinesia, the incidence of tardive dyskinesia was 1.0% with olanzapine and 4.6% with haloperidol.[318] There is also emerging evidence that olanzapine may possess an antidyskinetic effect, thus resulting in improvement in tardive dyskinesia among patients with pre-existing tardive dyskinesia.[319] Olanzapine is also less likely than either the typical antipsychotics or risperidone to induce hyperprolactinaemia.

However, olanzapine is associated with weight gain and metabolic disturbances during treatment.[282,320] The issue of weight gain is of concern because this is a widely used drug. Many patients gain some weight but a substantial proportion (perhaps 20–30%) of patients will become obese while on olanzapine. It has been suggested that weight gain may be associated with an enhanced response to olanzapine, but this is not clear. It has also been noted that patients receiving olanzapine may develop elevated cholesterol and plasma lipid levels, and a proportion may also show glucose intolerance and/or frank diabetes mellitus.[320] In the comparative study mentioned above,[317] these effects were similar in olanzapine-treated and clozapine-treated patients. Nevertheless, they are of concern. There is evidence that nifdizipine may reduce weight gain during olanzapine therapy.[321]

Quetiapine

Quetiapine is a dibenzothiazepine compound. It has a receptor binding profile that is broadly similar to that of clozapine.[268] Also like clozapine, studies with PET suggest that binding of quetiapine to dopamine D_2 receptors reaches a plateau (well under 50%) even when dosed up to the current maximum dose of 800 mg/day.[243] This may explain the virtual absence of EPS with this drug.[322] Kapur et al. have recently expanded this theory. They have shown that high D_2 occupancy occurs shortly after an oral dose of quetiapine, but that the drug does not persist in occupying the receptor because of its "fast dissociation constant".[323] This observation of the pharmacodynamic properties of quetiapine offers an elegant hypothesis that atypicality with these new drugs may (at least in part) be explained by a shorter period of binding to dopamine D_2 receptors. Further work is necessary to refine this hypothesis.

Quetiapine is typically prescribed at doses of 300–500 mg/day in the acute treatment of schizophrenia. Doses of 600 mg/day and above are generally required for maintenance therapy. Quetiapine is an effective antipsychotic for treating positive, negative and overall symptoms of schizophrenia.[324] In an 8-week trial in patients who were partial responders to prior treatment with a typical antipsychotic, 52% of quetiapine-treated patients responded versus 38% of the haloperidol-treated patients.[325] Quetiapine's efficacy on negative symptoms is superior to typical antipsychotics and similar to that of other atypical antipsychotics. Quetiapine reduces co-morbid mood symptoms in patients with schizophrenia.[326] Quetiapine can also enhance cognitive function in patients with schizophrenia and a study reported superiority of quetiapine over haloperidol in several cognitive measures.[327] There is no information on the effect of quetiapine on suicidality. There are some early data to suggest that quetiapine may be helpful for patients with schizophrenia who have persistent aggression.[328] However, its effect on acutely agitated patients is less well studied and there is no liquid or acute intramuscular form available as yet.

There is some initial information showing that quetiapine is effective and well tolerated as a first-line treatment for schizophrenia.[329]

"Quetiapine is typically prescribed at doses of 300–500 mg/day in acute treatment ... Doses of 600 mg/ day and above are generally required for maintenance therapy"

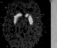
Quetiapine is also an appropriate choice for maintenance therapy.[330] There is some information on the use of quetiapine in treatment-refractory schizophrenia.[331] Clinicians are having experience with the use of quetiapine at doses beyond the recommended level of 800 mg/day, even at doses of 1200 mg/day, which appears to be well tolerated in these patients.[332]

Quetiapine has a particularly favourable side-effect profile with respect to EPS and a moderate profile with respect to weight gain and metabolic effects. Quetiapine is essentially devoid of EPS, even at high doses. Quetiapine is also substantially less likely than typical antipsychotics to cause tardive dyskinesia, with available data showing a very low 1-year incidence.[333] There is also no evidence of hyperprolactinaemia with quetiapine. There is evidence that quetiapine can cause weight gain, although this appears less pronounced than with clozapine or olanzapine.[334] Quetiapine has also been associated with diabetes mellitus.[335] There was initial concern (based on now considered overinterpreted pre-clinical information) that this drug was associated with cataracts, but post-marketing information does not confirm any excess in the frequency of cataracts.

At the time of writing, quetiapine is the most commonly prescribed antipsychotic in the USA.

Ziprasidone

Ziprasidone is an approved antipsychotic in the USA, but it is not yet available in the UK. It has a broad binding profile.[268] It is typically prescribed at doses of 80–160 mg/day, with 40 mg being the starting dose. There is emerging evidence for the benefit of higher doses (240 mg/day and above) of ziprasidone beyond the current recommended dose.[336] It is available in oral tablet and acute intramuscular forms.

Ziprasidone is effective for treating positive, negative and cognitive symptoms of schizophrenia.[337] Registration clinical trials showed that ziprasidone was statistically significantly better than placebo and comparable to haloperidol in reducing psychotic symptoms.[338] There is also evidence that ziprasidone can reduce cognitive deficits in patients with schizophrenia. There is evidence that ziprasidone can improve co-morbid mood symptoms and prosocial functioning in schizophrenia.[339] The effect of this drug on suicidality or on persistent aggression in patients with schizophrenia is currently unknown. However, ziprasidone is available in a short-acting intramuscular form and is an effective choice for the management of acutely agitated psychotic patients.[340]

Ziprasidone is well tolerated and has a favourable side-effect profile, especially with respect to EPS and also weight gain. Available

"Ziprasidone is typically prescribed at doses of 80–160 mg/day ... There is emerging evidence for higher doses (240 mg/day and above) beyond the current recommended dose"

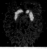

data from clinical trials suggest that ziprasidone causes minimal EPS, even when prescribed at high doses. There is little information on the incidence of tardive dyskinesia with ziprasidone. However, there is no reason to believe that the rate of tardive dyskinesia will differ substantially from the low rates that have been observed with the other atypical antipsychotics. Ziprasidone is noteworthy for causing less weight gain than (any of) the other atypicals.[282] In a short-term study in which patients were switched to ziprasidone from either typicals, risperidone or olanzapine, ziprasidone therapy was associated with a reduction in weight, particularly in patients who were previously on olanzapine.[341] Recent information on the 1-year follow-up of these patients shows pronounced weight loss in patients switched from olanzapine to ziprasidone.[342] Metabolic disturbances have also been shown to be less on this drug. In a recent study comparing 5 weeks of treatment with either ziprasidone or olanzapine, ziprasidone-treated patients had less weight gain, less glucose and insulin dysregulation, and lower lipid and cholesterol levels.[343] There was initial concern that ziprasidone may cause cardiac conduction irregularities, specifically prolongation of the QT_c interval on ECG. There are data from a study which compared the QT_c effects of several antipsychotics and only thioridazine was found to have a clinically meaningful effect on QT_c prolongation, causing rises above 460 ms.[344] On the other hand, it is recommended to avoid other risk factors (e.g. certain medications, low magnesium) for torsade de pointes during treatment with ziprasidone.

Aripiprazole

Aripiprazole is the latest antipsychotic to come on-line and is available for clinical use in the USA and in many European countries. Aripirazole is available in tablet, liquid and dissolvable tablet forms (tablet only in UK). An acute intramuscular formulation of aripiprazole is presently in an advanced stage of clinical investigation and may become available in clinical practice in due course. Aripiprazole has attracted considerable attention already because of its pre-clinical pharmacological profile (see Figs 64 and 65). It is considered to be a partial agonist at dopamine D_2 receptors, i.e. it binds to D_2 receptors with high affinity and acts as a functional antagonist in the hyperdopaminergic state and as a functional agonist in the hypodopaminergic state.[345–347] This apparently unique profile may confer an advantage of lower liability for EPS and hyperprolactinaemia. Additionally, aripiprazole has partial agonist effects at some serotonin receptors, notably at the $5-HT_{1A}$ subtype. It is also an antagonist at the $5-HT_{2A}$ receptor subtype. Collectively, it is proprosed that these effects can result in "neuromodulation" of the dopamine and serotonin systems. Therefore, the proposed mechanism of action of this drug is as a dopamine–serotonin system stabilizer.[347,348] It is important to observe, with the development of aripiprazole, how our conceptualization of the mechanisms of action of antipsychotic drugs has progressed beyond the initial idea of blocking overactive dopamine receptors.

There is information that aripiprazole is an effective and well-tolerated antipsychotic.[349–351] A placebo-controlled trial of 4 weeks' duration and including over 400 patients[349] compared aripiprazole (at fixed doses of 15 and 30 mg/day) with haloperidol (10 mg/day). Aripiprazole was superior to placebo on all primary symptom measures and was equivalent to haloperidol in improving symptoms. Aripiprazole was much better tolerated in terms of EPS and prolactin elevation than haloperidol. Another placebo-controlled study trial of 4 weeks' duration compared aripiprazole (at fixed doses of 20 and 30 mg/day) with risperidone (6 mg/day).[350] Both drugs were superior to placebo on all primary symptom measures and they appeared equivalent to each other in improving symptoms. Risperidone was associated with more EPS and prolactin elevation than aripiprazole. In another study, aripiprazole proved similar to olanzapine in efficacy but was associated with greater improvement on selective measures of cognition.[352] Aripiprazole is currently being studied; results to date are encouraging and of the same pattern as seen in the studies of intramuscular formulations of risperidone and of olanzapine.[353] There is preliminary evidence for the benefit of aripiprazole in patients with first-episode schizophrenia.[354] There is also evidence from a 1-year maintenance trial of aripiprazole versus haloperidol that aripiprazole has fewer relapses and is well tolerated.[355]

> *Aripiprazole is considered to be a partial agonist at dopamine D_2 receptors … This profile may confer an advantage of lower liability for EPS and hyperprolactinaemia*

There is one study of aripiprazole in treatment-refractory patients in which aripiprazole was similar in overall outcome (there was some benefit over perphenazine in quality of life) to the typical antipsychotic perphenazine.[356] Improvements in symptoms and on adverse effect parameters (especially in body weight) were observed in a study where patients were switched to aripiprazole from both typical and atypical agents.[357]

Aripiprazole has a favourable adverse effect profile. There is an absence of a dose-related increase in EPS, although the drug does appear to be associated with akathisia. This can be treated by lowering the dose of aripiprazole or adding a short-term course of a low dose of a benzodiazepine (or a beta-blocker). The drug has a favourable prolactin-sparing profile, findings that accord well with aripiprazole's proposed mechanism of action.[351] This drug also appears to be associated with a low propensity to cause weight gain, which may turn out to be a substantial advantage if confirmed in clinical practice. The cardiac profile of this drug also appears safe. Sedation appears to be the only dose-related side-effect, observed in approximately 10% of patients on 15 mg/day of aripiprazole

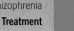

and about 15% of patients on 30 mg/day,[351] although the majority of responders from short-term trials (88%) did not experience somnolence. The drug can be given as a single daily dose, with a recommendation to commence at 15 mg, a dose which has been shown to be efficacious.

Sertindole

Sertindole is a phenylindole derivative atypical antipsychotic with a high functional antagonist affinity at dopamine D_2 receptors, serotonin receptors (specifically the 5-HT$_{2A}$ receptor subtype) and α_1 adrenergic receptors (see Fig. 68).[358,359] This appears, from electrochemical studies, to show a selectivity for inhibition of dopamine neurones in the ventral segmental region rather than those of the substantia nigral tract. This limbic selectivity may underlie its low liability for EPS and lack of pro-lactin elevation. Sertindole is now available for clinical use in several European countries, but is not presently available in the USA.

The results of a major, placebo-controlled trial of sertindole (at doses of 12, 20 and 24 mg/day) with haloperidol (4, 8 and 16 mg/day) confirmed that sertindole is an effective antipsychotic.[360a] The 20 mg/day dose of sertindole was the only dose of either drug to show superiority over placebo on negative symptoms. This has been confirmed in a recently published trial where sertindole has been shown to be superior to risperidone in reducing the PANSS negative symptoms.[360b] Sertindole has placebo level EPS and is generally well tolerated, apart from decreased ejaculatory volume.[361] A concern (which has also raised concern about antipsychotics as a class) has been QT_c prolongation and the risk of fatal cardiac arrhythmia.[362,363a] An extensive post-marketing surveillance study and careful reviews of all available information now suggests a cardiac profile for sertindole comparable to other antipsychotics. This data supports the current launch and increasing use of this drug in Europe.[363a] The effective dose of sertindole appears to be between 12 and 20 mg/day, with a starting dose of 4 mg/day. Furthermore, an exploratory trial suggests efficacy in treating the cognitive impairment in schizophrenia.[363b]

"The effective dose of sertindole appears to be between 12 and 20 mg/day "

Other "atypical" antipsychotic medications

Amisulpiride and sulpiride, both from the substituted benzamide class of drugs, are widely used in Europe (especially France) in the acute and maintenance treatment of patients with schizophrenia.[364] The extent to which these drugs can be considered atypical is unclear and it appears that their neurotransmitter receptor profile is predominantly dopamine D_2 blockade. This D_2 occupancy appears to be at rates that are more in line with typical than with atypical antipsychotic medications.[268] Also, both drugs are associated with EPS and tardive dyskinesia. On the other hand, there is evidence that these drugs may have superior efficacy over typicals, and they have been shown to be superior for treating negative symptoms of schizophrenia.[365]

Zotepine is an antipsychotic, which is best considered under the group of atypical antipsychotics. It is effective for treating positive, negative and cognitive symptoms of schizophrenia.[337] Clinical trials demonstrate that zotepine is superior to haloperidol in reducing psychotic symptoms.[366] There is also some evidence that zotepine improves cognitive functioning in patients with schizophrenia. Currently, there is insufficient information on the efficacy of zotepine for co-morbid mood symptoms, suicidality or aggression in patients with schizophrenia.

Zotepine has a good side-effect profile. It has low rates of EPS and has a low incidence of tardive dyskinesia. There is insufficient information on zotepine with respect to weight gain and metabolic disturbances.

Other medications used to augment the treatment response with antipsychotics

Optimizing monotherapy with the chosen antipsychotic is the preferred strategy

There is no obvious or 'best' choice of medication combination ... The choice is usually guided by the target symptom

Despite the availability of an ever-expanding range of typical and atypical antipsychotics, a substantial proportion of patients will show a partial or lack of response to antipsychotic monotherapy. Optimizing monotherapy with the chosen antipsychotic is the preferred strategy. Thereafter, most clinicians will choose an alternative antipsychotic as the next step in managing non-responders. However, there are several augmentation strategies that can also be tried. These include adjunctive antipsychotic medications (i.e. combining two atypicals or combining an atypical with a typical), mood stabilizers, selective serotonin reuptake inhibitors or glycinergic agents.[367–370] These options are highlighted in Fig. 69. The evidence for using augmentation strategies is not compelling and this approach is associated with only modest clinical improvement. Most experts would favour switching to another antipsychotic if the observed response is inadequate. Augmentation strategies are probably best restricted to the most severely ill patients who have not responded to other treatments. In general, there is no obvious or "best" choice of medication combination. The choice is usually guided by the target symptom – i.e. another antipsychotic for persistent positive symptoms, an antidepressant or mood stabilizer for co-morbid affective symptoms or a selective serotonin reuptake inhibitor for co-morbid obsessional symptoms. There is some evidence that "fish oil" may be a beneficial supplement to augment the response of antipsychotic medications; fish oil is not, however, considered a primary treatment for schizophrenia. There is also some preliminary evidence that hormonal therapy with oestrogen may enhance the response to antipsychotic medications.

Drug class	Target symptoms	Preferred choice
Antipsychotics • Typical • Atypical	Positive symptoms	Typical, e.g. haloperidol
Anticonvulsants • Valproate • Carbamazepine • Lamotrigine • Topiramate • Gabapentin	Positive symptoms; agitation/ aggression	Valproate
Benzodiazepines	Agitation/anxiety	Clonezapam
Glutamatergic agents	Negative symptoms	Glycine, D-cycloserine
Anticholinesterase inhibitors	Cognitive deficits	Donezepil
Antidepressants	Depressive symptoms	Selective serotonin reuptake inhibitors

Fig. 69 Adjunctive medications for the augmentation of antipsychotic response in schizophrenia

Non-pharmacological management
Electroconvulsive therapy (ECT)

The role of ECT in the treatment of patients with schizophrenia is limited (see Fig. 70).[371,372] ECT is indicated when a patient has a catatonic form of illness, a form of schizophrenia which is now considered rare. ECT is a treatment option when the patient has severe co-morbid depression. However, this is most often managed by antidepressant medications. ECT may be used when the depression is recurrent, severe and unresponsive to antidepressant treatments, and when it is associated with suicidality that is not diminished by antidepressant treatments. ECT is rarely used besides these indications of catatonia and severe co-morbid depression. It is best considered a treatment of last resort for patients with severe, refractory illness. It may be used safely with clozapine and other antipsychotic medications (see later section).

“ECT has a limited role”

Fig. 70 Use of electroconvulsive therapy (ECT) in the treatment of schizophrenia

Pattern of use
• was overused in the 1960s and 1970s when diagnostic rigour between schizophrenia and mood disorder was less clear
• now infrequently used

Indications for use
• catatonic subtype of schizophrenia
• marked co-morbid depression in schizophrenia, especially with suicidality
• refractory schizophrenia, when optimized medication therapy has failed

Psychotherapies (see Fig. 71)

There are a range of non-pharmacological, psychosocial and rehabilitative therapies that are effective in treating persons with schizophrenia.[373,374]

Individual

Supportive counselling/psychotherapy is an important aspect of the care of patients with schizophrenia.[375] This usually focuses on specific and daily activities, and it is not in the categories of classical or insight-oriented psychotherapy. There is ample evidence to indicate that the latter form of psychotherapy is detrimental and can result in relapse for patients with schizophrenia. However, this is often misconstrued to suggest that patients do not need or benefit from individual psychotherapy – this is simply an error. Patients have a tremendous need for

Fig. 71 Psychotherapeutic interventions in schizophrenia

Individual	Group	Cognitive behavioural
Supportive/ counselling	Interactive/social	Cognitive behavioural therapy (CBT)
Personal therapy		Compliance therapy
Social skillstherapies		
Vocational/ rehabilitation therapies		

support and counselling. There are many issues that are best treated with individual psychotherapy/counselling – the meaning and impact of psychosis, insight, individual goals and life expectations, relationships with family and friends, human intimacy and sexuality, career selection, stress management, etc. Recent research has attempted to define the core elements of psychotherapy and to ascribe specific forms, such as personal therapy (PT) or cognitive behavioural therapy (CBT). PT was developed by Hogarty and colleagues at Pittsburgh, USA.[376] It views affective dysregulation and stress management as the basic focus of therapy for patients with schizophrenia. PT attempts to enhance personal awareness of each stage of illness and to promote coping skills that are appropriate to the patient's status. Hogarty et al., in a 3-year study, reported that the relapse rate with PT was lower than the alternative treatment options of either traditional supportive psychotherapy or family therapy.[376] Recently, Hogarty and colleagues have reported on a further elaboration of their PT approach and find benefit for this in the care of people with schizophrenia.[377]

"Patients have a tremendous need for support and counselling"

Cognitive behavioural therapy

Cognitive behavioural therapy (CBT) in schizophrenia has been derived from its successful use in the treatment of depression.[378,379] This therapy had been adapted for application in patients with severe schizophrenia who experience persistent and distressing delusions or hallucinations. The techniques and competencies for using CBT in patients with schizophrenia are well described. Training in CBT is important because unilateral and confrontational challenging of a patient's chronic delusional system by an unskilled clinician may place the clinician at risk of harm and may also increase the risk of relapse for the patient. There are now several studies which confirm that this is an effective treatment. One study by Sensky et al. compared CBT with "befriending therapy" in patients with chronic schizophrenia.[380] Both treatment groups showed good outcome after 6 months of treatment; however, the effect was sustained in the CBT group, who had lower symptoms and better functioning 6 months after the treatment was discontinued. This treatment has also recently been used in the care of patients with schizophrenia following their first psychotic episode.[381] The results of CBT in this less ill group are encouraging. Another development is the use of CBT to enhance the patient's adherence with treatment – so-called "compliance therapy".[382] This approach attempts to utilize the patient's level of insight and appreciation of the risks and benefits of treatment to enhance the patient's commitment and compliance with therapy. There is evidence to support a role for this modality in the maintenance therapy of patients with schizophrenia.

"CBT to enhance the patient's adherence with treatment is called compliance therapy"

Family therapies

Family psychosocial therapies have arisen from the observation that patients who were stabilized on medication and then returned to families of high expressed emotion (HEE) experienced a poor outcome with relapses (see Fig. 72). Efforts to reduce this risk of relapse led to various psychoeducational and family therapy strategies.[373,374,383] Common themes that emerge in treatment with family members are listed in Fig. 73. There is a large body of literature which confirms that family psychotherapy using behavioural and psychoeducational techniques can achieve superior patient outcomes compared with routine care. Relapse rates are reduced with family interventions to about 25% compared with rates of 65% among patients who receive treatment as usual.

In addition, families have formed important self-help and advocacy groups such as SANE and NAMI. It is important that clinicians recognize that family involvement is a crucial component of treatment. Also, in the wake of a voluminous literature on HEE, it is important to appreciate that family interactions are not a cause of schizophrenia.

> *Family involvement is a crucial component of treatment*

Social skills training

Social skills training is recognized as an important treatment modality for patients with schizophrenia.[373,374,384] It is based upon behavioural and learning theory techniques. Social skills therapy focuses on the discrete components of social interaction that can be identified and targeted for intervention. It is recognized that, because of the early onset of this illness, many patients will never have learnt or experienced social situations (e.g. dating) that most adults have already performed and now take for granted. Social skills training also seeks to integrate, under a rehabilitation approach, the findings of cognitive (e.g. attentional) deficits and perceptual disturbances (e.g. impaired recognition of facial emotions), that diminish the patient's capacity for normal social interactions. Three broad approaches have been identified (see Fig. 74).

Fig. 72 Stress, family involvement and medication compliance

Patient variables		
Receiving medication	Contact with family	Relapse rate 9 months post-discharge (%)
Yes	Low expressed emotion	12
Yes	High expressed emotion, less than 35 hours contact per week	42
No	High expressed emotion, over 35 hours contact	92

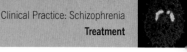

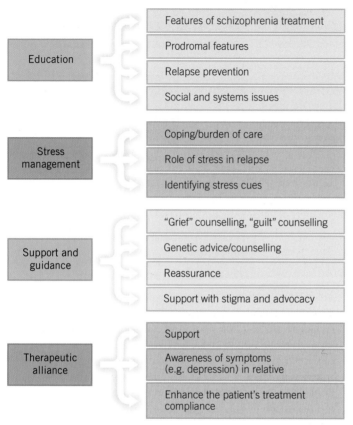

Fig. 73 Themes and components of family psychotherapeutic interventions

In the basic model, complex social repertoires are analysed and broken down into distinct steps. Each step is then role played and rehearsed until the patient has acquired the required skill. This approach has been shown to be effective, but it is not clear that these benefits transfer into community-living situations. In the social problem-solving model, role playing is augmented with various educational activities that aim to improve the attentional and information deficits of patients with schizophrenia. Modest benefits have been demonstrated with this approach.

The observation of cognitive deficits as a core feature of schizophrenia has prompted some recent research into cognitive treatment strategies for patients.[385] One current problem is the generalizability of response from cognitive remediation training to daily situations. A recent focus of interest has been the topic of "social cognition" in

Fig. 74 Social skills interventions in schizophrenia

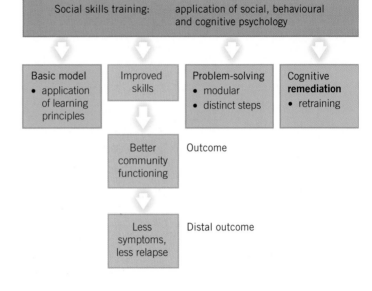

schizophrenia – that is, the capacity of patients to appreciate facial expressions (affective changes – anger, sadness, etc.) and to cognitively process these experiences and related social interactions.[386]

Case management

Case management (CM) is the provision of supportive personnel who assist the patient in daily living and disease management.[387–389] Allied mental health staff (e.g. community nurses, social workers or mental health "technicians") help patients to plan and attend social events, and to conduct routine tasks such as cooking, laundry and managing finances. Staff also accompany patients to outpatient visits and they will also oversee the patient's compliance with his/her prescribed medication. There are many forms of CM; generally, they vary in the intensity of service and in the patient-to-staff ratio. In the UK the Care Programme Approach (CPA) focuses on the need for a multidimensional care plan, regularly reviewed with the patient, and the provision of a key worker or care coordinator working within a multidisciplinary team. Assertive community treatment (ACT) is an important and well-studied form of CM.[387] The basic components of ACT are listed in Fig. 75. This approach has been shown to reduce the hospital relapse of patients and to maintain symptom control. To achieve functional and vocational goals, it is necessary to incorporate specific social and vocational strategies into the overall treatment plan. There has been considerable research in an effort to determine which is the most

• Outreach to patient – at home, in residential care
• 24-hour availability
• High staff : patient ratio, typically
• Frequent (daily/3–5 times per week) contact
• Coordinate all aspects of care – medical, psychiatric, social
• Functional performance and satisfaction (patient, family) are more important outcomes than symptom reduction

Fig. 75 ACT programme characteristics

appropriate and most effective CM model for patients and what type of personnel (e.g. nurses or technicians) are best suited to provide this form of "home care". In general, the service types are equivalent in outcome, and show improvements in re-hospitalization rates and overall quality of life. However, they have been less effective in getting patients back to work, which most consumers would consider an essential outcome measure.

Vocational rehabilitation
Vocational rehabilitation is a critical but most often under-resourced component of the comprehensive care of patients with schizophrenia. Only about 20% of patients achieve any form of employment and more often than not this is either sheltered employment or low-skilled and poorly paid work. Sheltered workshop and supportive work therapies have been shown to increase the quality of life and to sustain employment in patients.[390] However, rates of relapse remain high in these patients and unfortunately it is often only the least symptomatic patient who can withstand the stress of regular work without relapse. Bell and colleagues showed that a neurocognitive enhancement therapy added to work produced substantial improvements in cognitive function among patients with chronic schizophrenia.[391] Kurtz and colleagues also advocate the use of neurocognitive strategies to improve rehabilitation in persons with schizophrenia.[392]

Systems issues
Despite substantial treatment advances, we often provide care in mental health systems that is inadequately funded, poorly planned and often executed in a disjointed fashion. This has been the topic of a Presidential Commission on Mental Health in the USA, which concluded that the system needs to be "transformed" rather than (just) improved.[393] This is a major shift in thinking and takes account of the

❝To achieve functional and vocational goals, it is necessary to incorporate specific social and vocational strategies into the overall treatment plan❞

complexity of coordinating mental health, physical health, vocational, disability and social support services for people with severe mental illness whose needs are complex and necessitate good service integration. Thus, while this document focuses on the US healthcare system, the principles of service integration and coordination of care for patients with schizophrenia are relevant to all healthcare systems. There are often discontinuities between inpatient and outpatient care and across other aspects of services. Additionally, there is wide variability in the clinical practice. Patients may receive different medications based on the prescribing practices of psychiatrists rather than any clear distinctions in illness. There is sometimes disjointed care where, in spite of the availability and support for use of atypical antipsychotics, medications are switched too frequently and patients are exposed to periods of no treatment. In addition, there is considerable variability in the extent and quality of psychosocial and vocational services that are available to patients. There is also concern as to the "fidelity" of the practised model of service. For example, many services would claim to provide ACT, but when these services are evaluated with respect to the key elements of the ACT model they are found to fall short. Future directions in health services research and delivery will be to integrate social skills and assertive CM interventions with other approaches, such as vocational training, housing support, etc. The challenge to integrate our services is immense. Making real progress in treating schizophrenia requires attention to these many other needs, as well as providing availability to new medications. Integrating these components and tailoring these to the needs of the individual patients is the real challenge of comprehensive and continuous care for schizophrenia.

"The challenge to integrate our services is immense"

MANAGEMENT

Acute psychosis

The goals of acute management are:

- To conduct a careful assessment of symptoms and behaviour of psychosis.
- To evaluate and provide immediate management of the risk of suicide, if any exists.
- To evaluate and provide immediate management of the risk of harm to others, if this risk exists.
- To institute immediate measures to stabilize psychosis and to plan further care.

The acutely psychotic patient often presents in crisis (see Fig. 76). It is essential to conduct a thorough assessment in order to arrive at a presumptive or definitive diagnosis and also to plan for immediate care. Ruling out other conditions is an important first step of management

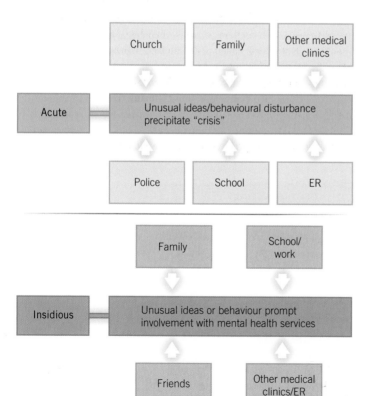

Fig. 76 "Pathways to care" for patients with first-episode psychosis

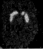
> **❝To plan for immediate care, it is essential to conduct a thorough assessment❞**

(see Fig. 77). As outlined earlier, a wide variety of general medical and central nervous system conditions can present with psychotic features that mimic schizophrenia. Additionally, psychotic symptoms related to substance abuse are often difficult to distinguish from schizophrenia. This circumstance may be further complicated by co-morbid substance abuse in patients who have a diagnosis of schizophrenia. Also, psychotic symptoms associated with schizophrenia may be similar to those seen in schizophreniform disorder, brief psychotic disorder, delusional disorder, schizoaffective disorder or bipolar disorder. Determining the correct diagnosis(es) is essential to treatment planning. Core aspects of the assessment of the acutely psychotic patient are highlighted in Fig. 78. The evaluation of risk of self-harm and harm to others is of particular importance. Alongside how florid the patient's psychosis is, these are the main reasons why a patient will be admitted to hospital as opposed to being cared for in a day hospital or in another outpatient setting.

The use of medications in the acutely psychotic patient are highlighted in Fig. 79. Acutely psychotic patients who are agitated will require immediate pharmacotherapy.[246] Every effort should be made to acquire informed consent to treatment from the patient. If medications are necessary and the patient consents, then medication treatment should be given in oral tablet, oral dissolvable (so-called "melt-in-your-mouth" tablets) or liquid form. Unfortunately, it is not uncommon for patients who present as acutely psychotic to deny their illness and, consequently, refuse medication (and often all other forms of treatment). At this juncture, the clinician is at an impasse and he/she must carefully weigh the immediacy and extent of risk against the competency and expressed wishes of the patient. When the risk of harm is immi-

Fig. 77 Other causes of first-episode psychosis which can resemble schizophrenia

- Organic brain disorders
  - head trauma
  - epilepsy
  - sarcoidosis
  - infections (HIV, encephalitis)
  - vasculitis (SLE)
  - multiple sclerosis

- Drug-induced psychotic disorder

- Brief psychotic disorder

- Mood disorder with psychosis

- Delusional disorder

Historical	Onset and duration of illness
• Rule out other aetiologies	Antecedent factors – head injury
• Confirm diagnosis	Substance abuse
	Medical history
	History from relative/close friend
Observational	Level of consciousness
• Rule out other aetiologies	Symptoms of psychosis
• Confirm diagnosis	Presence of mood features
• Evaluate treatment needs	Neurological evaluation
	Level of agitation
Ancillary	Laboratory tests
• Rule out other aetiologies	• Haematology
• Confirm diagnosis	• Metabolic
• Support treatment planning	• Drug and alcohol
	Neuroimaging
	Detailed collateral information, including assessment of carers' needs

Fig. 78 Assessment of the patient presenting with a first psychotic episode

Option	Management
Antipsychotic	Low dose to minimize potential for side-effects; use more sedating drug if agitation is a problem; use acute intramuscular preparation if risk to self/others
Benzodiazepine	Use – not routine; use if agitation; use intramuscular preparation if agitation is a substantial problem
Chloral hydrate	Use – not routine; use if agitation or insomnia

Fig. 79 Choice of medication interventions in the acutely psychotic patient

nent and serious, immediate action is required and the patient should be involuntarily medicated. In this (unfortunate) circumstance, medication must be given in intramuscular form.[394] One choice for medications by the intramuscular route are typical antipsychotics and/or a short-acting benzodiazepine. The advantage is that these agents work and are inexpensive. The main disadvantage is the substantial risk of inducing EPS, especially acute dystonia, which is damaging to the therapeutic alliance at such a crucial stage. Now that atypical antipsychotics are increasingly becoming available in short-acting intramuscular and in dissolvable forms, clinicians are beginning to use these more as the preferred option for managing acute agitation.[395]

If the risk of harm is serious but less immediate – and the patient still refuses treatment – then the clinician must decide whether to commit the patient to hospital against his/her will.[396] The procedures and legal requirements for involuntary commitment differ substantially from country to country.

If the risk of harm is low but the patient is in need of continued observation because of the degree of psychosis, then the clinician must decide whether hospitalization or day treatment is appropriate. This will depend on many factors, chief of which are the extent of the patient's psychosis (especially the amount of behavioural control and insight the patient exhibits) and the extent of support the patient has.

First-episode psychosis

Patients may present acutely, with florid psychotic symptoms, or they may come to treatment after a long and insidious onset of illness; the latter is associated with poorer treatment response and poor long-term outcome. The importance of a thorough assessment at the beginning of treatment cannot be emphasized enough. Although clinicians differ on the extent of medical evaluation at the onset of psychosis, most would consider it prudent to order some routine biochemical and imaging tests (see Figs 5, 6 and 78).

There is no clear choice of any particular antipsychotic as the first-line treatment. In Europe, clinicians often commence therapy using one of the typical antipsychotics, although this practice is changing rapidly. In the USA, clinicians now prescribe an atypical antipsychotic as the first-line treatment. This is consistent with treatment guidelines. As is the case with the typicals, there is no guidance (as of yet) as to which of the atypical agents is the best option. It is likely that the atypical agents are essentially equiefficacious in this highly responsive population and at present there are no direct comparative studies published to inform clinical practice.

Studies of risperidone, olanzapine, quetiapine and aripiprazole in first-episode schizophrenia have been described in an earlier section. It is important to appreciate that patients experiencing their first episode of psychosis are at a stage of illness that is, in general, more responsive than later to medication and other treatments.[397] They are also much more sensitive to the adverse effects of medications. For both reasons, clinicians usually begin treatment with low doses of the chosen antipsychotic medication. In the acute, hospital setting, the medication may be increased every 2–3 days depending on tolerance and response. With this approach, one can expect to reach an appropriate maintenance dose in a matter of days.

On the other hand, if the patient is less psychotic and is being treated as an outpatient, then the escalation of dose will be slower and will occur typically over the course of several weeks. In either instance, it is critical that the patient and clinician be alert for the emergence of side-effects. Failure to recognize and effectively treat adverse effects in first-episode patients leads to non-compliance with therapy; this will ultimately result in a relapse of psychosis. The adage "start low and go slow" is useful when initiating antipsychotic therapy in this group.

It is also critical to provide supportive psychotherapy/counselling during (and after) this first episode of psychosis. Aspects that are the focus of therapy at this stage are highlighted in Fig. 80. CBT has also been shown to be an effective treatment at this stage of the illness.[381]

"Failure to recognize and effectively treat adverse effects in first-episode patients leads to non-compliance and ultimately relapse of psychosis"

Education	Features of schizophrenia
	Treatment options
	Prodromal features and relapse prevention
	Social support and information on resources, disability support, with focus on recovery
	Tackling drug misuse
Role clarification and outcome expectations	"Grief" counselling
	Clarification of likely short-term, intermediate treatment outcomes
	Functional, social, occupational goal setting
	Reintegration

Fig. 80 Themes and components of counselling for the first episode of psychosis

Maintenance therapy

Effective maintenance treatment can decrease the frequency and the severity of the episodes of illness, reduce its morbidity and mortality, and maximize the psychosocial functioning and the quality of life of patients. While some patients have an excellent outcome and therefore only need periodic monitoring, most patients require comprehensive and continuous care over the course of their illness.

With regard to medication treatments, the benefit of maintenance pharmacotherapy must be balanced against the risk of long-term side-effects of treatment.[235] The positive impact of typical antipsychotic medications on the course of illness has been highlighted earlier. These drugs reduce relapse and can improve functioning. Their main drawback in long-term therapy is the risk of tardive dyskinesia. This risk can be minimized by using the lowest effective dose of the typical antipsychotic medication (see earlier section) and by switching to an atypical antipsychotic if EPS occurs and/or if there is early evidence of tardive dyskinesia. The lower risk of tardive dyskinesia, in combination with a broader efficacy profile, are reasons why atypicals are used for maintenance therapy. There is now growing information on the longer-term efficacy and in particular comparative trials of atypical antipsychotics. The favourable results of the 1-year relapse prevention study of risperidone versus haloperidol were described earlier. There are now direct comparative trials of risperidone versus olanzapine, of risperidone versus quetiapine, of olanzapine versus quetiapine, of olanzapine versus ziprasidone, and of ziprasidone versus risperidone. In a 28-week double-blind study, patients receiving risperidone and patients receiving olanzapine improved over time.[398] There was evidence for superiority of olanzapine over risperidone with respect to the amelioration of depressive and negative symptoms. The olanzapine-treated patients also had generally fewer side-effects. However, not unexpectedly, the olanzapine-treated patients experienced more weight gain (4.1 ± 5.9 kg versus 2.3 ± 4.8 kg). This study was conducted shortly after both risperidone and olanzapine became available in clinical practice and the dosing profiles (mean modal doses: olanzapine, 17.2 ± 3.6 mg/day; risperidone, 7.2 ± 2.7 mg/day) are unbalanced, particularly the dose of risperidone, which is in excess of current dosing in clinical practice. In a smaller and more naturalistic 6-month follow-up study[399] of patients being treated with either risperidone (6 mg/day) or olanzapine (14 mg/day), both drugs proved comparable in efficacy during the first 4 weeks of acute treatment, but risperidone proved superior for overall amelioration of psychotic symptoms at 6 months. Another 8-week, double-blind prospective trial compared risperidone (mean modal dose of 4.8 mg/day) with olanzapine (12.4 mg/day) in patients with chronic schizophrenia.[400] Risperidone-treated patients showed a greater improvement in positive and anxiety/depression symptoms. Rates of EPS were comparable between both drugs. More weight gain occurred in the olanzapine group. A recent study of olanzapine versus quetiapine favoured olanzapine in efficacy, but there was also more weight gain in olanzapine-treated patients.[401] There is also information on the comparative efficacy of risperidone and quetiapine. A 4-month open-label trial[326] of quetiapine (mean dose 254 mg/day) versus risperidone (mean dose 4.4 mg/day) in patients with psychotic disorders (almost 75% of patients had a diagnosis of either schizophrenia or schizoaffective disorder) revealed that both drugs were efficacious across a range of symptoms. There was a slight advantage for quetiapine in treating depressive symptoms. Quetiapine was also associated with less EPS. Another recent comparison of quetiapine and risperidone showed similar efficacy,[402] while another study favoured risperidone, which was also associated with less polypharmacy.[403] A study of ziprasidone versus olanzapine has been described – the drugs

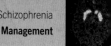

were similar in efficacy, with better tolerability seen for ziprasidone.[343] A recent short-term comparative study between ziprasidone and risperidone showed similar overall outcomes in efficacy, but better tolerability with ziprasidone.[404]

In the absence of convincing and substantial comparative trials of each atypical antipsychotic in refractory schizophrenia, choice of medication in this patient group is, in part, being influenced by their relative adverse effect profile. The adverse effect profile of antipsychotic medications is a major issue in the maintenance treatment of schizophrenia. It has been argued that atypical antipsychotics are better tolerated than typicals and that this is a major justification for favouring atypicals for long-term management. However, the emergent side-effect profile of atypicals (weight gain, metabolic complications) is worrisome, particularly for long-term management.[405] There is now substantial concern about atypicals inducing weight gain and metabolic disturbances and their serious long-term health consequences.[284,406] In a 5-year report of 101 patients who had been treated with clozapine for at least 1 year,[290] weight gain was maximal during the first year of treatment, but patients continued to gain weight up to month 46. Of considerable concern is the high rate (52% at the end of 5 years) of new-onset diabetes mellitus. There was a non-significant increase in total serum cholesterol and a significant increase in triglycerides. In another study[320] of weight gain and metabolic disturbance in patients treated, on average, for 6 months with olanzapine (median dose of 12.5 mg/day), 57% of patients had a Body Mass Index above normal, 20% had hyperglycaemia, 71% had elevated insulin levels, 62% hypertriglyceridaemia, 85% hypercholestrolaemia and 57% had elevated leptin levels. Summaries of the current understanding of antipsychotic-induced weight gain and of metabolic complications are given in Figs 81 and 82.

> **❝Most patients require comprehensive and continuous care ❞**

> **❝The benefit of maintenance pharmacotherapy must be balanced against the risk of long-term side-effects of treatment ❞**

Is a major concern in treatment, requiring pre-counselling and informed consent before initiating antipsychotic treatment
Can occur on all antipsychotics, although some are more likely than others
Pattern is more of visceral adiposity, which of itself predisposes more to metabolic complications
Identifying weight gain early in treatment and intervening is critical
Although various medications (antiobesity drugs) and behavioural interventions may help, most clinicians opt to switch to another antipsychotic of (hopefully) lower weight gain liability
Research on pharmacogenetic risk for weight gain may turn out to be helpful in predicting which patient on which drug will gain

Fig. 81 Synopsis of current understanding of weight gain during antipsychotic therapy

Fig. 82 Synopsis of current understanding of metabolic disturbances during antipsychotic therapy

Is a major concern in treatment, requiring pre-counselling and informed consent before initiating antipsychotic treatment
Can occur on all antipsychotics, although some are more likely than others
Risks include developing diabetes mellitus, hypertriglyceridaemia, hypercholesterolaemia and the metabolic syndrome
Genetic and other demographic and health factors are probably of greater significance than medication in determining who is predisposed to these metabolic complications
Evaluation of risk factors, thorough pre-treatment evaluation and ongoing monitoring are key components of treatment
Most clinicians opt to switch to another antipsychotic when metabolic complications arise

This is an area of intense research, and hopefully breakthroughs in understanding and in intervention will emerge to counteract the risks of these drugs. At the present time, while clozapine and olanzapine seem to be the two drugs most associated with weight gain and metabolic disturbances, it is important to stress that these effects can be seen in patients taking any of these new agents – the risk is only relative, with ziprasidone and aripiprazole currently showing the least propensity to cause these effects. Accordingly, given that these effects are associated with use of these drugs "as a class" (even though there appear to be real within-class differences in tolerability), new standards have been proposed to guide how best to screen patients and implement monitoring for weight gain, diabetes mellitus and other metabolic disturbances. These are highlighted in Fig. 83. These also call for specialist referral and ideally co-management of patients between psychiatrists and internal medicine specialists. It is less clear what – and when – are the most appropriate treatment intervention studies for managing weight gain, diabetes mellitus and other metabolic disturbances. The most frequent approach in practice today is to switch a patient to another agent once these adverse effects become problematic.

> **These guidelines also call for specialist referral and ideally co-management of patients between psychiatrists and internal medicine specialists**

The potential for cardiac effects of antipsychotic medications is another issue in the long-term management of schizophrenia. The topic of cardiotoxicity of antipsychotic medications, in particular QT_c prolongation and the risk of torsades de pointes, is complex and its clinical relevance in the care of the majority of patients is unsure at present.[362,406–408] There have been reports of fatal myocarditis–cardiomyopathy and pulmonary embolism during clozapine therapy.[282,283] It is now considered prudent to obtain an ECG at regular intervals (see Fig. 83) in patients on maintenance pharmacotherapy with antipsychotic medications.

Obtain baseline personal and family history of risk factors
Obtain baseline weight, height and vital signs measurements
Obtain ECG if indicated
Obtain baseline fasting blood glucose, lipids and cholesterol
Measure weight, height and vital signs regularly during treatment
Measure fasting blood glucose, lipids and cholesterol periodically during treatment
Obtain ECG periodically during treatment (frequency currently is much debated)

Fig. 83 Evaluating and monitoring for weight gain and metabolic disturbances during antipsychotic therapy

Several key points can be made about the maintenance pharmacotherapy of schizophrenia. First, treatment response remains highly individualized and although there is ample evidence that each of the antipsychotics described above is effective in treating schizophrenia, it is difficult in an individual patient to predict whether one drug or another will prove effective. It is hoped that the new research direction of pharmacogenetics may in time provide better predictive ability.[409] Second, while there is emerging evidence for class superiority of atypical over typical antipsychotic medications in the maintenance therapy of schizophrenia, there are as yet too few data to distinguish with any confidence treatment differences between each of the atypical agents. Where differences emerge, it is typically with respect to the side-effect profile of these drugs. Third, it is exceedingly common (in approximately 30% of patients in the USA) for patients to be treated with various combinations of medications – either a typical antipsychotic with an atypical, two atypicals together, an antipsychotic plus a mood stabilizer, an antipsychotic plus a benzodiazepine, or any combination thereof (Fig. 84).[410,411] The merits of this practice and the optimum choice of polypharmacy are presently unknown. Fourth, because we have had a spate of new antipsychotics in recent years, we are still very much in a learning phase with respect to the optimum dosing and duration of clinical trials of each drug. Therefore, there is wide variability in clinical practice with respect to how long a trial and at what dose of agent a patient will be treated with before changing to another drug. Inevitably, this gap in knowledge and the variability in treatment leads to frequent switching between these drugs.[412] This itself is a major issue. Guidelines for switching from one drug to another are given in Fig. 85.

The focus of psychological support during maintenance therapy needs to be broad and also individualized to the patient's needs. Issues of relevance to counselling may range from acquiring friendship, interviewing for part-time employment, to human sexuality.[375] The clinician needs to possess the same skills and empathy for the patient's

105

Fig. 84 Rational polypharmacy in schizophrenia

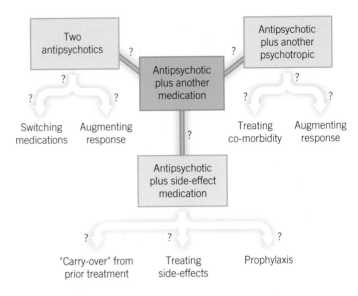

Fig. 85 Switching from one antipsychotic to another

Risks	Somatic withdrawal symptoms
	Relapse of psychosis
Management	Avoid "cold turkey"
	Cross-taper
	• gradual phase-out of first medication
	• gradual increase of new medication
	Avoid leaving the patient "stranded" on two drugs

dilemmas as he/she might for any other patient that is more "high functioning". CBT may help to reduce delusions and hallucinations, although this modality is best practised by a skilled clinician.[380] This approach may also be used to enhance the patient's long-term compliance with therapy, so-called "compliance therapy".[382]

Treatment-refractory schizophrenia

Despite optimum care, a substantial proportion of patients (perhaps 30%) will fail to show an adequate response to treatments.[314] These patients with treatment-refractory (TR) schizophrenia constitute the most difficult to treat group. They are also the patients who are disproportionate users of the mental health (emergency and legal) services.

Clozapine is the treatment of choice for TR schizophrenia. This is confirmed in several studies and key meta-analyses (see "Prevention" section). As yet, there is insufficient information on the comparative

Agent	Efficacy
Typical antipsychotics	"By definition" ineffective
Clozapine	Effective in possibly 60% of patients
Risperidone	Effective, but less so than clozapine
Olanzapine	Effective, probably less so than clozapine, although some data show comparability
Quetiapine	Efficacy at high doses, but extent is undetermined at present
Ziprasidone	Efficacy at higher doses
Aripriprazole	Undetermined at present
Sertindole	Comparable efficacy to risperidone in only refractory study available
Zotepine	Undetermined at present

Fig. 86
Pharmacotherapy of "treatment-refractory schizophrenia"

efficacy of clozapine and the other atypical antipsychotics. Available studies are conflicting and difficult to interpret, in part because of variable definitions of treatment resistance. On balance, these currently point to clozapine's advantage in severe TR schizophrenia. On the other hand, they also show that some TR patients will respond to other atypical antipsychotics (see Fig. 86).

Information on the use of other atypical antipsychotic medications is emerging. There is evidence that this drug is effective in a proportion of refractory patients.[413] For olanzapine, Breier et al. have analysed data on patients with TR schizophrenia (*n* = 526) who were a subgroup of the multi-centre comparative trial of olanzapine versus haloperidol.[414] In a last observation carried forward analysis, olanzapine-treated patients showed greater response rates than haloperidol-treated patients (46% versus 35%). On the other hand, Sanders and Mossman found that only two of 16 patients with severe schizophrenia/schizoaffective disorder showed a significant response to olanzapine.[304] The evidence for quetiapine, ziprasidone and aripiprazole has been covered earlier.

Which medication (i.e. which drug in what order, and when) sequence is the best is still very unclear. Available treatment guidelines do not distinguish one atypical from another. On current evidence, there seems to be no defined rationale for starting with one drug instead of the other. Also, which drug to try next is unclear, and at present this choice is largely driven by patient preference and an appreciation of the relevant side-effect profile of each drug. It is still unclear how long you should wait on one drug before switching to another

"Despite optimum care, a substantial proportion of patients have inadequate responses to treatments"

"Which drug to try next is unclear, and choice is largely driven by patient preference and drug side-effect profile"

66A 6- to 8-week trial of an antipsychotic is recommended – longer if the dose of medication was too low 99

drug. The decision depends on several factors, particularly the extent of response and the extent of side-effects that the patient is experiencing on his/her present medication. Usually, it is recommended that a patient receives a 6- to 8-week trial of an antipsychotic. This may need to be longer if the dose of medication was too low. On the other hand, the trial might be appropriately aborted before 8 weeks if the patient experiences distressing or serious side-effects. It is generally considered that a longer trial period (probably about 4 months) is required to adequately assess a patient's response to clozapine.

At what time point the clinician should resort to clozapine therapy is also unclear. Clozapine is under-utilized in the USA and Europe, in part because clinicians have relegated it to the treatment of last resort, after trials of several of the atypical antipsychotics. In one study of refractory patients with prior exposure and inadequate response to risperidone, haloperidol and then olanzapine, 50% of patients then responded to a trial of clozapine.[415] This observation is important because it confirms the clinical impression that failure to respond to one atypical antipsychotic does not preclude response to another agent. However, we still lack clear guidance as to the appropriate sequence (and dose) of trial of each agent and when, if warranted, to proceed to clozapine therapy.

What to do when clozapine therapy fails is a real dilemma.[368] One approach is to try adding in several agents to augment the response to clozapine. These approaches are more of a trial-and-error process. In one recent study, glycine, an N-methyl-D-aspartate (NMDA) receptor agonist, was added to clozapine therapy in 27 patients with schizophrenia.[416] There was no observed benefit to adding glycine, in contrast to the beneficial effect of NMDA agonists in augmenting response to typical antipsychotic medications.

ECT is another treatment option for patients with refractory schizophrenia who have failed other treatment options. A recent literature review of ECT augmentation of clozapine response suggests that 67% of patients benefit from augmentation with ECT. Adverse effects (prolonged seizures, non-fatal cardiac arrhythmias) occurred in 17% of patients.[372] ECT should only be considered for treatment-refractory patients following a careful review of prior treatments and after a second opinion has been obtained from another psychiatrist.

Cognitive behavioural therapy (CBT) may also be helpful for persistent delusions.[374,378,379] In one study, refractory patients received CBT or supportive counselling. Both groups improved during the 9 months of therapy. However, the CBT group continued to improve beyond the treatment period.[380] CBT is a useful modality, but its cost-effectiveness needs to be determined. ACT is another important intervention.[388]

Co-morbidities
Depression and suicide

Depression is common in patients with schizophrenia.[417] At least 50% of patients become depressed at some stage during their illness. Depression is associated with more frequent relapses and with a poorer outcome. Depression in schizophrenia is also associated with suicide. It is critical for mental health professionals to appreciate this close association and to be of heightened awareness of the risk of suicide in patients with schizophrenia who exhibit signs of co-morbid depression.[418] It is reliably estimated that approximately 50% of patients attempt suicide at some point during their illness. Awareness of the factors that may contribute to suicide among people with schizophrenia and the early detention of and intervention with people who are at risk for suicide are key components for successful management. There is also emerging information suggesting a positive impact of present-day pharmacotherapy on suicidality in schizophrenia.[419] The main element of this work concerns the atypical antipsychotic clozapine and several studies show that, through some yet to be elucidated mechanism, clozapine appears to exert an antisuicidal effect in people with schizophrenia.[420] The largest and most recent investigation is the International Suicide Prevention Trial (InterSePT).[276] This was a multi-centre, randomized controlled trial comparing clozapine with olanzapine treatment in 980 patients with schizophrenia or schizo-affective disorder who were at high risk for suicide through previous attempts or their current mental state. Suicidal behaviour over a 2-year period was reduced by almost a quarter in the clozapine group, with similar reductions in suicidal behaviour and associated hospitalizations.

Potential mechanisms for this antisuicidal effect may include a (direct) thymoleptic effect, an enhancement of insight (either directly and/or indirectly through improved cognition), or enhanced quality of life on this medication such that the patient is not overwhelmed by the hopelessness of intractable illness. An antisuicidal effect of clozapine (and perhaps other atypical antipsychotics) is an intriguing proposition and is consistent with heightened treatment expectations that extend beyond amelioration of symptoms to ultimately more profound domains of outcome in schizophrenia, specifically suicide and aggression.

"Depression is associated with relapses and poorer outcome, particularly with suicide"

Violence

The public perception and understanding of schizophrenia is that most patients are likely to be violent and that patients have a "Jekyll and Hyde" predisposition for violence. This is grossly misleading and wildly overestimated. Although rates vary widely depending upon the population studied and the definition of violence, approximately 15%

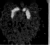

of patients with schizophrenia exhibit violent behaviour.[421] Active psychosis is a prominent risk factor for violent behaviour in schizophrenic patients and, although there are some associations between particular symptom constellations (the "threat–control override" pattern), the evidence for distinct symptoms as risk factors is less pronounced than one might intuitively consider. Substance abuse is also a major risk factor for the occurrence of violence in schizophrenic patients. Non-compliance with medication, inextricably linked with an active co-morbid substance and with psychotic decompensation, is another prominent risk factor.[422–424] A prior history of aggressive behaviour and of being abused as a child are other risk factors. At the same time, however, since risk factors such as substance abuse, acute psychotic decompensation and command hallucinations are all too common features in the course of schizophrenia, it is hardly surprising that these are, at best, only modest gauges of the imminent risk of violence – arguably the strongest clinical predictor. The prediction of imminent risk of violence is heightened by the closer temporal relationship to prior violence, the presence of signs of acute agitation and actual threats of violence.

The pharmacological management of the acutely agitated/aggressive patient has been covered earlier.

The pharmacological management of persistent aggression in patients with schizophrenia is complex. Because such patients are often non-compliant with treatment, they are appropriate candidates for a trial of a long-acting intramuscular antipsychotic. However, their illness is frequently unresponsive to standard treatments and these patients often receive multiple medication combinations. These combinations are changed frequently on a trial-and-error basis. There is emerging evidence that clozapine may be a particularly effective treatment for schizophrenic patients with persistent aggression. Beyond medication, the management of their care is more complex because it brings social and legal issues to the fore. The management of the patient with schizophrenia who has a history of violence constitutes a careful balance between the patient's clinical/personal needs and the perceived risk of violence for the community at large, i.e. societal needs. Since control of illness is a key principle of managing the risk of violence, then contentious treatment options, such as forced medication or involuntary hospitalization, must be considered.[425] These approaches are, to a large extent, logical from a clinical perspective of risk management – particularly given the accruing evidence that risk of violence is interrelated with level of disease activity – but they juxtapose serious ethical and social concerns that already have a long and inglorious history in the care of people with serious mental illness.

> *"Public perception that patients have a 'Jekyll and Hyde' predisposition for violence is grossly misleading"*

> *"The management of the violent patient requires a careful balance between the patient's clinical/personal needs and the perceived risk of violence for the community at large"*

Co-morbid substance abuse

Substance abuse co-morbidity (SA) in schizophrenia is a major concern, both in view of the frequency of SA among patients with schizophrenia and the notorious difficulty in managing such patients. The ECA study reported a prevalence of SA at 47% among patients with schizophrenia.[426] The consequences of SA in schizophrenia are extreme. These patients are much greater users of psychiatric services. In addition, they are seen more frequently by the emergency services and are more likely to use jail services. Available evidence suggests that the long-term course of SA in patients with schizophrenia is poor, both in terms of the persistence of SA and the poor outcome in substance-abusing patients. Elements of comprehensive care are outlined in Fig. 87. Treatment programmes emphasize many of the 12-step approaches that are advocated in the treatment of primary alcoholism and SA. In addition, they emphasize the development of social skills, behavioural management and motivational enhancement therapy.[427] The pharmacological management of SA in schizophrenia is less well studied. There are emerging clinical data to suggest that atypical antipsychotics, particularly clozapine, may be beneficial in the management of patients with co-morbid substance abuse and schizophrenia.[428]

> **These patients are much greater users of psychiatric, emergency medical and jail services**

Co-morbid obsessive-compulsive symptoms with schizophrenia

Obsessive-compulsive symptoms, co-morbid with schizophrenia, occur in approximately 5–7% of patients.[429] Although the presence of obsessive-compulsive disorder (OCD) symptoms was thought to predict a better outcome, these features typically characterize a poor outcome and intractable symptoms. It is unclear as to how to treat these symptoms and there is evidence that these features can uncommonly emerge de novo during treatment with an atypical antipsychotic medication. Selective serotonin reuptake inhibitors have been tried, but their use is complicated by their effect of elevating the plasma level of the antipsychotic. Given such a pharmacokinetic interaction, these drugs should be used with caution during clozapine therapy.

> **Obsessive-compulsive symptoms occur in approximately 5–7% of patients**

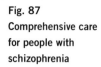

Fig. 87
Comprehensive care
for people with
schizophrenia

1. Best practices pharmacotherapy
Is dynamic
Reflects current literature
Is consistent with established standards of care
Needs to be integrated with other services/supports
Can synergize with other modalities

2. Responsibilities of the clinician in prescribing antipsychotic medications
Clinicians need to discuss:
• risks and benefits
• side-effects
Should have leaflets and educational handouts available

3. Setting goals for medication treatment
Specific
Measurable
Consistent with standards of care
Consistent with established outcome expectations
"Stable on current medications" may be too low an expectation of treatment outcome

4. Establishment of a strong continuum of care for best practices pharmacotherapy
Clinicians need time, support and resources to communicate effectively with other clinicians. These resources include:
• clear documentation of medications
• appropriate sharing of documentation and prescription details
• clinician-to-clinician discussion of medication treatments

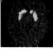

FUTURE DEVELOPMENTS

The pace of new drug development for schizophrenia is exciting and offers hope to patients and their relatives. Several drugs are at advanced stages of development. These new drugs represent refinements of current proposed mechanisms of drug action and/or new mechanisms (Fig. 88). For example, bifeprunox, currently at the advanced stage of clinical drug development, is a drug that has a similar receptor binding profile to aripiprazole. It has been shown in early studies to be an effective antipsychotic.[430]

Neural system	Focus/effect
Dopamine receptors	Partial agonist – antagonism Highly selective antagonist
Serotonin receptors	Highly selective antagonist (with or without dopamine antagonism)
Sigma receptors	Antagonist
Glutamate receptors	Agonist/antagonist
CNS phospholipid metabolism	Omega-3 fatty acid supplements
CNS oestrogen receptors	Oestrogen

Fig. 88 New mechanisms of action of putative novel antipsychotics/antipsychotics under development

There is also interest in examining the role of sigma receptor antagonists, GABA agonists and other highly selective agents in the treatment of schizophrenia. There is also substantial interest in the role of antioxidants in the treatment of schizophrenia, this work being based upon the findings of phospholipid abnormalities in patients with schizophrenia.[431] At present, these approaches are experimental and are not recommended for clinical practice.

There is also interest in the role of pharmacogenetics to enhance the prediction of patient response to antipsychotic medications.[409] In one study,[432] six polymorphisms of serotonin receptor genes were highly predictive (with a sensitivity of 95%) of a response to clozapine. Other studies have shown an association between alleles of serotonin receptor subtypes and the risk of weight gain. There is also some evidence of an association between dopamine receptor polymorphisms and antipsychotic-induced hyperprolactinaemia.[433] This focus of research has substantial potential and clear relevance for the management of schizophrenia and it raises the (currently far-off) possibility that we

❝Pharmacogenetics may enhance the prediction of patient response and tolerability to antipsychotics❞

113

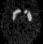

may in the future be able to individualize treatment regimes. There is also growing interest in the treatment of cognitive deficits in schizophrenia.[434–436]

There is also a more general trend in the USA toward greater integration of mental health and medical care for people with schizophrenia.[437] It is increasingly being recognized that patients with schizophrenia have high rates of physical co-morbidity and that this clinical dilemma may be further complicated by the medical effects (obesity, diabetes mellitus, cardiotoxicity) of the atypical antipsychotic medications. Consequently, there is an emerging trend towards greater involvement of other medical specialists in the care of people with schizophrenia. In the UK, the move to integrate mental health and social care may mitigate against this.

There is also evidence that the management of schizophrenia will be increasingly influenced by the evidence-based medicine (EBM) approach.[438,439] This will be of assistance in providing the context for appropriate pharmacotherapy, as well as ensuring that health care systems provide the full range of services (ACT, case management, vocational support) that are of proven effectiveness in the long-term care of people with schizophrenia (Fig. 89).

Finally, there is growing appreciation of the inherent capacity of individuals to recover from their illness. This paradigm, growing in prominence in the USA, emphasizes the person's own mastery over their treatment and refocuses the treatment plan on goals that are specific and meaningful for the patient (rather than symptom reduction,

❝There is growing appreciation of the individual's capacity to recover from illness ❞

Fig. 89 Evidence-based medicine (EBM) and schizophrenia

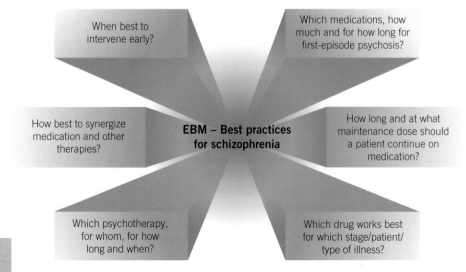

When best to intervene early?

Which medications, how much and for how long for first-episode psychosis?

How best to synergize medication and other therapies?

EBM – Best practices for schizophrenia

How long and at what maintenance dose should a patient continue on medication?

Which psychotherapy, for whom, for how long and when?

Which drug works best for which stage/patient/ type of illness?

which is generally a key focus for the clinician). There is interest in extending the role of peer support services, wherein people recovering from mental illness help others make progress in their treatment goals. This recovery-based approach has been a much valued and successful component of Alcoholics Anonymous (including the so-called "sponsor") for more than three decades now. While the recovery model is intuitively appealing and is an approach that is likely to grow in momentum, it also needs to be rigorously studied in the care of persons with schizophrenia.

"People recovering from mental illness can help others make progress in their treatment goals"

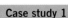

Case study 1
First-episode schizophrenia

History

Eddy is 24 years old. He worked as a mechanic until recently, giving up his job out of the blue, saying it was a waste of time. He did reasonably well at school, was sociable and positive in his outlook, last year proposing marriage to his girlfriend. He smoked cannabis occasionally at weekends, but used no other drugs and didn't drink alcohol. His parents are divorced and he lives with his mother. Her boyfriend, with whom she has a long-term and stable relationship, has recently moved in.

Over the last 6 months Eddy's mother has noticed that he has become increasingly introverted. He stopped going out and no longer returns his friends' calls. He has lost his appetite over the past month and has obviously lost weight. His fiancée has left him, saying she was fed up with him being depressed and moody all the time.

Eddy has told his mother that he is concerned for her safety, but he would not explain further. When questioned about his concerns he became upset and angry. At other times he has shut himself in his room. She has heard him talking angrily, sometimes shouting; he denies this.

His uncommunicativeness, anger and suspiciousness have gradually increased, and things came to a head one evening when he became agitated and smashed the mirror in the sitting room, cutting his hand. He was so agitated and distressed that his mother's partner felt it necessary to restrain him physically; Eddy got a black eye in the process.

His paternal uncle has a history of schizophrenia, and his father has been described as isolated and "a loner".

The following day, Eddy's mother attended her primary care centre and expressed her concerns. She has been unable to persuade him to come and see the doctor, who agreed to visit. When he did, he could not gain access to Eddy, who locked himself in his room, and would only answer "I'm alright, go away" to all questions.

The physician arranged an emergency multidisciplinary assessment with the local psychiatrist. At this visit Eddy reluctantly emerged from his room, and seemed frightened and agitated. He was initially unwilling to discuss the events of the previous evening, but eventually admitted that he felt he had to smash the mirror because it was the door to another frightening world from which he felt electric currents entering his spine and thereby controlling his stomach and bowels.

He is convinced that he and his mother are in terrible danger, and is unsure whether his mother's boyfriend is part of a conspiracy against them emanating from this place. He has heard voices describing his bodily functions, though did not wish to elaborate. At times these voices have spoken directly to him, threatening him with damnation, and he admits it is this that has frightened him and caused him to shout when isolated in his room.

Diagnosis

This man appears to have first-episode schizophrenia, though further assessment will be necessary. The history of withdrawal, apathy and depression during the previous 6 months represent a classic prodromal syndrome, with these features becoming overshadowed by positive psychotic symptoms and the behavioural response to them. It is likely that these psychotic symptoms include Schneiderian first-rank symptoms with somatic hallucination, delusions of control and third-person voice hallucination describing some of his actions.

It is possible that this presentation may represent a depressive psychosis, but the evolution of the prodrome and characteristics of the psychosis make this less likely than schizophrenia; a mixed syndrome is possible. It seems unlikely that this is due to drug intoxication, is otherwise related to substance abuse, or secondary to an organic cause other than schizophrenia. Nevertheless, a urinary drug screen is the most important investigation and he should have a physical work-up, including a neurological examination and special investigations, as necessary.

In terms of cause, it is likely that there is a genetic diathesis with schizophrenia in a paternal uncle (though the diagnosis should be confirmed, if possible), and the possibility of schizotypy, a schizoid or even paranoid personality disorder in his father. Triggering factors are less clear here, but the possibility of stress at home with mother's new live-in boyfriend should be taken into account. Whether it was a trigger will never be clear, but it may be an important factor in his rehabilitation and future accommodation.

Management

Regarding treatment, this is a pretty hot clinical situation that could easily lead to further violence and compulsory admission. However, much of Eddy's behaviour may be explicable in terms of his psychosis, including his weight loss and concern over his mother. Having got him talking, a good mental health team may be able to engage him over the coming days and weeks, and put a community care plan in place. A brief admission would be usual here because of the difficulties at home. He needs an antipsychotic drug fairly promptly, probably an atypical, but this could be started in a low dose to avoid immediate side-effects, with agitation being controlled with a regular benzodiazepine in the short term. People in their first psychotic episode are exquisitely sensitive to effects and side-effects of antipsychotic drugs, and a toxic experience can put someone off this important treatment for life; care is required.

He has a mixture of good and bad prognostic features. His DUP is fairly short, probably about 4 weeks, though his illness has been evolving for about 6 months. His pre-morbid function seemed pretty good, though being male with a family history of schizophrenia is not on his side. His age at onset is around the mode. The most important thing is to find an antipsychotic drug that suits him, and for Eddy to stay on it, rather than stop it when he feels better; psycho-education and cognitively-based compliance therapy may be useful therapeutic allies. He should do quite well but needs careful treatment, rehabilitation and follow-up.

Treatment-resistant schizophrenia

History

Matt Briggs is 37 years old and has just registered with the health centre. The previous notes are not available, but a recent hospital letter was faxed in advance. Matt was diagnosed at the age of 26 as suffering from paranoid schizophrenia. He had a history of substance abuse, including cannabis, LSD, ecstasy, cocaine and amphetamines. His illness had a gradual onset over a period of 2 years, including growing suspiciousness, withdrawal from his family and social networks, and loss of his job, culminating in an acute psychotic breakdown. At the time of his breakdown he suffered from an elaborate delusional system, including the belief that he was a "Messiah". He was admitted to a mental hospital in London under section 2 of the Mental Health Act. This was changed to a section 3, and he spent a total of 8 months in hospital, the last two as a voluntary patient. According to the letter, his symptoms have always been difficult to control, and he has already had treatment with trifluoperazine, chlorpromazine, thioridazine, pimozide and a year on depot flupenthixol, during which he relapsed. All have been at therapeutic doses.

He presents with a request for your advice on his medication. He has, until recently, had some contact with the community mental health team in his area, and has had a reasonable relationship with a community psychiatric nurse. However, he has never been enthusiastic about his antipsychotic medication and has stopped taking it on at least three occasions in the past 10 years. Each time he has ended up in psychiatric hospital. He is now on oral haloperidol (10 mg, three times a day) and an anticholinergic drug.

He wants to stop taking his medication again and wonders what you think about this.

He has the mask-like face and slow movements of drug-induced Parkinsonism. He is restless and shows evidence of akathisia. There is some evidence of facial involuntary movement.

When you question him more closely about his reasons for wanting to stop taking medication he begins to become excited. He points out, quite reasonably, that the physical side-effects of the medication are difficult for him to tolerate. He argues that the medication is acting as a barrier between him and his mission to the people. He believes that he has been sent on this mission by a higher power. When you ask him what the mission consists of, he replies that he must spread the truth, and speak to people about their lives and what they really need. He feels he cannot do this as long as he is taking antipsychotics, as they are blocking his thoughts and preventing the message getting through to him. He is not experiencing auditory hallucinations, and seems to want to engage in a discussion with you.

Management

There are still many people who have stories like this, slipping through the net as they move from place to place, driven partly by psychosis, partly by cognitive and social decline, partly by thoughtless decisions by those who should be helping them. Matt's schizophrenia has always been difficult to treat, and fulfils any criteria for treatment resistance. He has had trials of several antipsychotics at full dose and, furthermore, he relapsed on a depot so it's not about compliance; even now he's talking to you about his medication even though, clearly psychotic, he doesn't like it.

Psychiatrists may have focused more on his behaviour than his symptoms, and initial trials of antipsychotics were undertaken before second-generation or atypical drugs were widely used; some of his drugs we no longer use routinely. Whether wittingly or not, he's been marooned on ineffective drugs that keep him quiet through their side-effects; the Messiah causes much less trouble with a Parkinsonian syndrome and other EPS. However, this is entirely unacceptable and may even drive him to suicide; akathisia is a particular risk, as is ongoing psychosis. What Matt needs is a trial of clozapine and some hard work from a rehabilitation team.

To get clozapine, Matt needs prompt referral to a psychiatric team who will need to undertake a careful assessment; Matt wouldn't be the first person with chronic mania to be misdiagnosed, but he almost certainly has schizophrenia. They will need to make a good case to him to try the drug and accept the routine blood monitoring. This will be difficult and it is quite unclear whether he will be able to take a truly informed decision. Compulsory admission under Mental Health Act legislation should be considered, even though Matt has sought help. He's never had the best treatment, by the sound of it, and deserves a try.

He has several adverse prognostic features but his psychosis may resolve on clozapine, and his quality of life is likely to improve without the burden of extrapyramidal and other side-effects from the first-generation drugs. The possibility of an emergent orofacial dyskinesia is another indication for this drug. Nevertheless, he'll experience new side-effects on clozapine, and needs warning about, amongst others, the dribbling, sedation, transient enuresis, sedation and possibly worsening of cardiovascular risk factors that probably aren't great already; clozapine's side-effects go far wider than its rare effects on the white blood cell count, and need careful management to get the most out of this very effective drug.

Even if there is a beneficial effect, it is rare that chronic delusional systems such as this evaporate completely; people have lived with them for a long time. More likely, the psychosis will bother him less and less, he'll get on with life and will increasingly talk about things in the past tense. One day, he may feel it's over or that he made a mistake, but that's not very common in this situation. Some people do not respond to clozapine and have a new disorder, "clozapine-resistant schizophrenia", something that needs an expert team, often going back to basics, in the first instance.

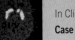

Case study 3

Chronic schizophrenia

History

Mrs Philodopolous is 68 years old and lives with her husband, who is 10 years her senior. She has had a number of psychotic breakdowns in her life. These began when she was in her mid-30s, after she had been married for 10 years. She has been admitted to mental hospital on a number of occasions, sometimes as a voluntary patient, sometimes under compulsion. She has been treated with a number of antipsychotics in her life, including chlorpromazine, haloperidol, thioridazine and finally settling on depot medication, flupenthixol decanoate (80 mg, administered every 2 weeks), at her primary care centre. None of these treatments have ever entirely abolished her psychotic symptoms, although they have been effective to different degrees in reducing her agitation and distress.

Mrs Philodopolous initially presented with thought insertion and broadcast, intensely distressed that sexual thoughts put into her mind by a neighbour were available to anyone in her house, who would look down on her and think she was dirty because of their content. She felt she was responsible for the thoughts and tried to resist them. She kept her house spotlessly clean so as to suggest to her neighbours and friends her pure heart and good housekeeping, and was very anxious at the thought of dirt that would confirm these people's negative views of her. By her second admission and consistently since, she had a delusional system which includes the belief that she has been visited by an unknown man during the night who sexually assaults her while she and her husband sleep; she thinks she may be pregnant. Mr and Mrs Philodopolous have never had children.

Until 5 years ago she had been attending a psychiatric outpatient clinic regularly, every 6 months. She had been under the care of the same consultant psychiatrist for over 20 years. After his retirement she had stopped attending outpatients. She had become increasingly withdrawn and suspicious, and had refused to leave her house over the last 4 months. During this period she had stopped attending her GP's surgery for her depot medication, so this had been administered by a community psychiatric nurse who visited the home.

Her husband, who suffers from chronic obstructive pulmonary disease, has become increasingly unwell during this period and is less able to care for her. He seems less tolerant of her, and appears exhausted. In response to this she has withdrawn from the sitting room to her bedroom, and her delusion of pregnancy has become stronger, and increasingly preoccupies her thoughts. She has shouted in the night that she is in labour on more than one occasion. An increase in the dose of the depixol has not produced any improvement in her mental state. Unfortunately, she has developed Parkinsonian-type adverse effects on the higher dose.

Diagnosis

Mrs Philodopolous' case is, in some ways, similar to Matt's chronic delusions in the context of paranoid schizophrenia in Case study 2, but there are interesting and important differences spanning the neurobiology and social formulation of these cases.

The initial presentation here, with phenomenology reminiscent of obsessive-compulsive disorder, reminds us of the fact that these syndromes may coexist. Some people, say about 5%, have OCD symptoms or something akin before the onset of schizophrenia when the symptoms resolve, and a similar number get the problem as the schizophrenia evolves. The OCD symptoms in schizophrenia are often not as clearly ego-dystonic as in operational definitions of the disorder. Rather they are somewhere on a spectrum between ego-alien and ego-dystonic phenomena and may have links to other psychotic symptoms; here, they are towards the former end. This coexistence is presumably due to basal ganglia dysfunction in both schizophrenia and OCD. The symptoms are often difficult to treat in schizophrenia, requiring dopamine blockade or modulation from antipsychotics that are being taken anyway, the addition of a specific serotonin reuptake inhibitor (SSRI) and cognitive behavioural therapy. Prognosis is not good.

The domestic situation is not good in this case. One has to admire the marriage, having stayed strong through some difficult and probably humiliating circumstances, but it seems under great strain now. It may be that this strain and increased expressed emotion has triggered an exacerbation of Mrs Philodopolous's symptoms; it certainly won't be helping. On the other hand, one should also think of other triggers and, in older age, physical illness may be an important trigger.

Mrs Philodopolous needs a complete physical health screen when considering her decline; something such as hypothyroidism, vitamin B12 or folate deficiency could be the key and easily remedied. People with schizophrenia are just as vulnerable to independent physical conditions as are others, perhaps more so, for some illnesses. A new, though more rare, syndrome such as a cerebral tumour, likely a secondary, should be borne in mind, just as it should in someone without schizophrenia.

Cognitive decline and dementia also need to be ruled out. The relationship between schizophrenia and dementia is not straightforward. Cognitive function is almost always affected even before schizophrenia, with some covert effects present even in childhood. Cognition is profoundly affected by onset of psychosis but there is probably a variable course thereafter, this course partly determining functional outcome. It is uncertain whether schizophrenia is an independent risk factor for an independent, new dementia in old age, but it may be. Just as psychosis may be part of the Alzheimer syndrome, so there may be an exacerbation of psychosis if cognition declines, whatever the cause.

Common things being common, a careful drug history should be taken, as these may be contributing to cognitive decline. Here, one may need to look no further than the anticholinergic effect of Mrs Philodopolous's antipsychotic drugs.

Management

There are dilemmas in how best to help this couple, and whether to be apparently heavy-handed by precipitating their separation and rehousing separately. These will need careful consideration. However, in the short term, aggressive investigation, reformulation of Mrs Philodopolous's change in mental state and reconsideration of treatment, perhaps as an inpatient, and the same for her husband's lung condition, may restore the status quo for a while, and allow the couple to live together again, for a while at least. If this is not possible, the difficult decision about separate accommodation needs to be faced, but in the knowledge that the quality of their relationship may remain good if the separate accommodation is suitable, and there are means to support them seeing each other. Others will take a different view, and the couple's own thoughts should be central.

Case study 4
Schizophrenia in pregnancy

History

Davine Salmond is a 32-year-old professional woman. She has had two psychotic breakdowns with a florid paranoid schizophrenia syndrome, and on both occasions has been admitted to psychiatric hospital. She has responded very well to antipsychotic drugs during these admissions. The second breakdown occurred when she had stopped her medication because she thought she was cured.

She has no psychotic symptoms at present. She has a good network of support from friends and family. She lives with her mother, who has sickle-cell anaemia, and her maternal grandmother. Her maternal grandfather has schizophrenia and learning difficulties; her father is reported to have had bipolar disorder but is no longer on the scene and the diagnosis is unconfirmed.

Davine was fostered for brief periods in her childhood when her mother was unwell and required hospital admission. She and her grandmother are now the carers for the mother when she becomes unwell with sickle crises. She has a job as an office manager and publicity officer for a national charity, and has a steady relationship with her boyfriend, who she has been seeing for 3 years. She has no children.

Her current medication is risperidone depot (Risperdal Consta; 25 mg every 2 weeks). She has been quite happy with this for at least 2 years. You and she have discussed stopping the drug on a few occasions, but the memory of her last breakdown is very frightening for her, and neither you nor she are keen to alter the status quo.

She tells you that her last period was 10 weeks ago and that she has confirmed an unexpected though not unwanted pregnancy with a test she has bought at the chemist's. She has discussed her pregnancy with her partner and her family, and she has decided she wants to have the baby. She has three worries that she wants to talk to you about. The first, and most pressing, is whether it is safe for her to continue with the medication during pregnancy. She is very worried that the medication might harm the growing baby. The second, related concern is whether she is more likely to have a breakdown in or immediately following pregnancy anyway. Her grandmother has implied that this is the case. The third is her concern that her child might inherit her vulnerability to psychotic disorder.

Management

This situation has many strands, and the patient, Davine, has identified some of the most important. The most immediate concern is the continued management of her schizophrenia and the risk to the foetus. Davine has already proven that she needs antipsychotic medication to stay well, and that her recovery is profound with excellent occupational, personal and social functioning. Her current medication suits her. On the other hand, she does not wish to expose the foetus to drugs. There is a lot to put at risk on both sides of the equation.

For any drug, at any time, the benefits have to outweigh the risks. We would recommend that Davine continues on the risperidone, but that she should not breast-feed. Others may take a different view, and the exact licensing of the drugs in any country may be a factor.

The risk to the foetus, in terms of potential teratogenesis, would, as with any drug, be greatest during the first trimester; this pregnancy is almost through that period. However, the absolute risk is small. It seems entirely reasonable, and would be part of her proper antenatal care, for Davine to have expert obstetric assessment, ultrasound scanning and counselling regarding what to do in the unlikely event that an abnormality is detected – this may or may not have anything to do with her antipsychotic, of course.

She may consider changing her antipsychotic to one such as chlorpromazine, where there is great experience during pregnancy and where the risk to the foetus is defined as being very low through accumulated experience. However, Davine may not respond well to this drug, and the crossover period would be difficult.

The main period of increased risk in terms of relapse of her psychosis is in the final trimester and the first 2–3 months after the birth. Relapse can occur despite treatment, so a care plan identifying early signs of relapse and what to do if they occur should be in place.

Having said that, a relapse signature that includes common components such as sleeplessness, lack of concentration and irritability may not be very discriminating for first-time parents soon after the birth – everyone gets these features to a degree. She needs careful monitoring and support, as does the family. Who, for instance, will care for the mother if she has a sickle crisis and Davine is busy with the baby? A plan for relapse needs to include the baby, the family and, if possible, liaison with a perinatal psychiatry team, perhaps with access to inpatient facilities suitable for mothers and babies.

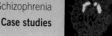

The risks to the child fall into several categories. Maternal bonding and early development of the child are certain to be affected if Davine relapses; this is why relapse prevention is so important. Extrapyramidal effects in the neonate have been reported occasionally with antipsychotics, and the child would need monitoring; liaison with a paediatrician may be best done through the perinatal psychiatry team. As mentioned, continued exposure through breast-feeding is not advised.

In terms of genetic risk of schizophrenia, the baby certainly has an elevated risk with an affected mother and maternal great-grandfather, and may have an affected grandfather too. We would put it to Davine that her baby has around a one-in-four to one-in-five chance of developing schizophrenia or another major psychiatric disorder. This is quite high but, on the other hand, Davine knows that recovery is entirely possible, and better treatments and understanding are coming on stream. When her child moves into the period of risk, after puberty, who knows what may be available in terms of early diagnosis and treatments, perhaps even prevention.

Case study 5
The great imitator

History

Jayne Treveux is a 49-year-old fashion shop manager, married with two young children. She was referred to a local psychiatrist by her primary care physician having been suspended from work after complaints from customers that she was offering them spiritual rather than sartorial advice, and insisting they read passages from the Bible before she would help them choose clothes. Her colleagues complain that she spends all her break times praying, and her husband and children say she has been increasingly obsessed with religion over the past 6 weeks, believing that they should attend church daily or they will be taken by the devil and killed; she thinks various orbiting satellites have been placed there by Satan in order to monitor the piety of all US citizens. Prior to this, she had had no particular religious beliefs, describing herself as an atheist.

A detailed history showed several episodes over this same period where she had woken from a nap with a headache and having been incontinent, something quite new for her. She wasn't bothered by this, though noticed that she had lost weight and felt tired and worn down by her responsibilities to the world.

On examination, Jayne presented as a relaxed middle-aged woman who spoke in a verbose manner on religious themes, but who had a range of other conversation. There was no evidence of an emotional or anxiety disorder and no hallucination. She had fixed beliefs about satellite monitoring of the USA, as above. Interestingly, she felt she knew this must be happening because of the smell of incense she experienced at the height of her prayer.

A working diagnosis of paranoid schizophrenia was made and she was started, as an outpatient, on an atypical antipsychotic at adequate dose. Compliance was good with family support.

Six weeks later, the picture had worsened, and she presented as an emergency having been found unconscious. She had been praying in a corner of a room for up to 12 hours per day, thinking this was the only way to destroy the power of the evil satellite system and save mankind. Over the past week there had been several periods of up to 5 minutes where she had appeared completely preoccupied, moving her lips rhythmically, staring into the middle distance and responding to no stimuli. She had told her husband that she had heard the voice of God retelling her thoughts behind her.

On the day of presentation, her husband had returned to find her lying on the floor. There was bleeding from her mouth and she had been incontinent. Physical and neurological examination was normal otherwise. The diagnosis was of increasing psychosis with intense religious preoccupation leading to neglect of bodily functions. She was admitted to hospital. The dose of antipsychotic was increased.

She was found dead in bed the following morning. Post-mortem examination showed signs of asphyxia as the cause of death, consistent with death in the context of epilepsy. A small breast carcinoma was present, with several metastatic deposits in the left frontal and temporal lobes of the brain.

Comments

Few professionals will see this kind of picture of focal temporal lobe seizure with generalization and signs consistent with a space-occupying lesion. It's easy after the event; little was typical about this presentation but nothing was inconsistent with the working diagnosis.

Jayne was quite old for a first-episode psychosis, though still within the conventional range, particularly for women. Religiosity is said to be associated with temporal lobe pathology, though all and any feature of schizophrenia, including first-rank symptoms, may occur in temporal lobe epilepsy.

The weight loss and systemic features, the history that was strongly suggestive of epileptic seizures, in retrospect at least, and the atypical psychotic features may have rung alarm bells. The psychosis worsened with treatment with antipsychotics, rather than getting better, almost certainly reflecting the reduced seizure threshold. This paradoxical worsening of psychosis should have made one think of epilepsy.

The key learning point here is the importance of the conventional full history and examination as part of the initial assessment: mental state and physical state. This may have picked up the tumour.

A full assessment should also include EEG and, where possible, structural brain CT or MRI; either would most likely have identified the secondary tumours.

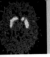

DRUGS USED TO TREAT SCHIZOPHRENIA

Drugs used to treat schizophrenia

Drug	Trade name	Preparation	Starting dose (mg/day)	Usual dose range for maintenance (mg/day)	Maximum dose (mg/day)
Clozapine	Clozaril leponex	Tablet	12.5–25	150–600	900
Risperidone	Risperdal	Tablet, liquid	1–2	3–6	16
Olanzapine	Zyprexa	Tablet, dissolvable wafer	5–10	10–20	20
Quetiapine	Seroquel	Tablet	50–100	300–600	800
Ziprasidone	Zeldox/Geodon	Tablet	40–80	40–160	160
Aripiprazole*	Abilify	Tablet	10–15	10–30	30
Pimozide	Orap	Tablet	2	2–20	20
Haloperidol	Haldol	Tablet, liquid	1–5	5–25	60
Haloperidol decanoate	Haldol-D	Long-acting injection	25–50 (IM)	50–200/2–4 weeks	300/3–4 weeks
Trifluoperazine	Stelazine	Tablet, liquid	2–5	2–20	20
Zuclopenthixol	Clopixol	Tablet	20–30	20–50	150
Zuclopenthixol decanoate	Clopixol-D	Long-acting injection	50–100	200–400/2–4 weeks	600 weekly
Chlorpromazine	Largactil	Tablet, liquid	50–100	300–800	1000
Thioridazine	Melleril	Tablet, liquid	50–100	300–800	800
Thiothixene	Navane	Tablet, liquid	5–10	15–50	50
Loxapine	Loxitane	Tablet	20	50–100	150
Perphenazine	Trilafon	Tablet, liquid	4–8	16–56	64
Molindone	Moban	Tablet, liquid	20	50–100	150

*No European licence at present

130

Drugs used to treat schizophrenia

Drug	Trade name	Preparation	Starting dose (mg/day)	Usual dose range for maintenance (mg/day)	Maximum dose (mg/day)
Fluphenazine	Prolixin	Tablet, liquid	5	5–20	20
Fluphenazine decanoate	Prolixin D	Long-acting injection	12.5–25	12.5–50/2–4 weeks	100/4 weeks
Zotepine	Zoleptil	Tablet	50–75	150–300	300
Sulpiride	Dolmatil	Tablet	400–800	800–1600	2400
Amisulpride	Solian	Tablet	400–800	400–800	1200
Sertindole**	Serdolect	Tablet	4	12–20	24

**Only available in Europe on restricted basis only

ABBREVIATIONS

Abbreviations	
ACT	assertive community treatment
CBT	cognitive behavioural therapy
CM	case management
COMT	catechol-O-methyltransferase
CT	computerized tomography
DLPFC	dorsolateral prefrontal cortex
DUP	duration of untreated psychosis
DZ	dizygotic
EBM	evidence-based medicine
ECT	electroconvulsive therapy
EPS	extrapyramidal side-effects
fMRI	functional magnetic resonance imaging
GABA	γ-aminobutyrate
HEE	high expressed emotion
5-HT	5-hydroxytryptamine
Ig	immunoglobulin
MRI	magnetic resonance imaging
MZ	monozygotic
NMDA	N-methyl-D-aspartate
NMS	neuroleptic malignant syndrome
OCD	obsessive-compulsive disorder
OR	odds ratio
PET	positron emission tomography
PT	personal therapy
QT_c	QT interval (corrected for heart rate)
QTL	quantitative trait loci
SA	substance abuse co-morbidity
SPD	schizotypal personality disorder
SPET	single photon emission tomography
SSRI	specific serotonin reuptake inhibitor
TR	treatment refractory

USEFUL WEBSITES

Cambridge Early Intervention in Psychosis (CAMEO)
www.cameo.nhs.uk

Expert consensus guidelines on schizophrenia
www.psychguides.com

Harvard Psychopharmacology Algorithm Project
www.mhc.com/Algorithms

Mental Health Infosource
www.mhsource.com
www.mentalhelp.net

National Alliance for the Mentally Ill (NAMI)
www.nami.org

National Institute for Clinical Excellence
www.nice.org.uk

Rethink (National Schizophrenia Fellowship of United Kingdom)
www.rethink.org

SANE
www.sane.org.uk

Schizophrenia home page
www.schizophrenia.com

WPA site on Stigma Campaign Against Schizophrenia
www.openthedoors.com

www.mental-health-matters.com

www.mentalhealth.com

www.mentalwellness.com

www.planetpsych.com

www.psyweb.com

REFERENCES

1. Andreasen NC. Symptoms, signs and diagnosis of schizophrenia. *Lancet* 1995;**346**:477–81.
2. Harrison G, Hopper K, Craig T, et al. Recovery from psychotic illness: a 15- and 25-year international follow-up study. *Br J Psychiat* 2001;**178**:506–17.
3. Murray RM, Lewis SW, Reveley AM. Towards an aetiological classification of schizophrenia. *Lancet* 1985;**i**:1023–6.
4. Susser MW. *Causal Thinking in the Health Sciences. Concepts and Strategies in Epidemiology.* New York: OUP, 1973.
5. Kendell RE. Schizophrenia: the remedy for diagnostic confusion. *Br J Hosp Med* 1972;**8**: 383–90.
6. Clare A. *Psychiatry in Dissent: Controversial Issues in Thought and Practice.* Tavistock, UK, 1979.
7. Zubin J, Spring B. Vulnerability – a new view of schizophrenia. *J Abnorm Psychol* 1977;**86**(2):103–26.
8. American Psychiatric Association. *Diagnostic and Statistical Manual of Mental Disorders*, 4th ed. Washington, DC: American Psychiatric Association, 1994.
9. World Health Organization. *The ICD-10 Classification of Mental and Behavioural Disorders: Diagnostic Criteria for Research.* Geneva: World Health Organization, 1993.
10. International Early Psychosis Association: http://www.iepa.org.au/.
11. McGorry PD. The recognition and optimal management of early psychosis: an evidence-based reform. *World Psychiat* 2002;**1**(2): 76–83.
12. Mason P, Harrison G, Glazebrook C, et al. The course of schizophrenia over 13 years. A report from the International Study on Schizophrenia (ISoS) coordinated by the World Health Organization. *Br J Psychiat* 1996;**169**:580–6.
13. Shepherd M, Watt D, Falloon I, et al. The natural history of schizophrenia: a five year follow up and prediction in a representative sample of schizophrenics. *Psychol Med* 1989;**15**(Monograph Suppl):1–46.
14. Steadman HJ, Mulvey EP, Monahan J, et al. Violence by people discharged from acute psychiatric inpatient facilities and by others in the same neighborhoods. *Arch Gen Psychiat* 1998;**55**:393–401.
15. Buckley PF, Hrouda DR, Friedman L, Noffsinger SG, Resnick PJ, Camlin-Shingler K. Insight and its relationship to violent behavior in patients with schizophrenia. *Am J Psychiat* 2004;**161**:1712–4.
16. Heaton RK, Baade LE, Johnson KL. Neuropsychological test results associated with psychiatric disorders in adults. *Psychol Bull* 1978;**85**:141–62.
17. Green MF. What are the functional consequences of neurocognitive deficits in schizophrenia? *Am J Psychiat* 1996;**153**:3.
18. Häfner H, Maurer K, Loffler W, et al. The influence of age and sex on the onset and early course of schizophrenia. *Br J Psychiat* 1993;**162**:80–6.
19. Kirkbride J, Fearon P, Morgan C, et al. Heterogeneity in incidence rates of schizophrenia and other psychotic syndromes: findings from the three-centre ÆSOP study. *Arch Gen Psychiat* 2005, in press.

20. Kraepelin E. Dementia praecox. In: *Psychiatrie*, 5th ed. Leipzig: Barth, 1896; pp. 426–41. Translated in: Cutting J, Shepherd M. *The Clinical Roots of the Schizophrenia Concept*. Cambridge: CUP, 1987; pp. 13–24.

21. Bleuler E. Die Prognose der Dementia Praecox – Schizophreniegruppe. *Allg Z Psychiat* 1908;**65**:436–64. Translated in: Cutting J, Shepherd M. *The Clinical Roots of the Schizophrenia Concept*. Cambridge: CUP, 1987; pp. 59–74.

22. Bleuler E. *Dementia Praecox oder Gruppe der Schizophrenien*. Leipzig, Vienna: Deuticke, 1911.

23. Weinberger DR. Schizophrenia: from neuropathology to neurodevelopment. *Lancet* 1995;**346**:552–7.

24. Erlenmeyer-Kimling L, Cornblatt B, Friedman D, et al. Neurological, electro-physiological and attentional deviations in children at risk of schizophrenia. In: Henn FA, Nasrallah HA, editors. *Schizophrenia as a Brain Disease*. New York: OUP, 1982; pp. 61–98.

25. Fish B. Infants at risk for schizophrenia: sequelae of a genetic neurointegrative defect. *Arch Gen Psychiat* 1992;**49**:221–35.

26. Fish B. Neurobiological antecedents of schizophrenia in children. *Arch Gen Psychiat* 1977;**34**:1297–313.

27. Walker E, Lewine RJ. Prediction of adult-onset schizophrenia from childhood home movies of the patients. *Am J Psychiat* 1994;**147**:1052–6.

28. Marcus J, Hans SL, Auerbach JG, et al. Children at risk for schizophrenia: the Jerusalem infant development study. *Arch Gen Psychiat* 1993;**50**:797–809.

29. Wadsworth MEJ. Follow-up of the first national birth cohort: findings from the Medical Research Council National Survey of Health and Development. *Paediat Perinatal Epidemiol* 1987;**1**:95–117.

30. Wadsworth MEJ. *The Imprint of Time. Childhood History and Adult Life*. Oxford: Clarendon Press, 1991.

31. Jones PB, Harvey I, Lewis SW, et al. Cerebral ventricle dimensions as risk factors for schizophrenia and affective psychosis: an epidemiological approach to analysis. *Psychol Med* 1994;**24**:995–1011.

32. Crow TJ, Done DJ, Sacker A. Childhood precursors of psychosis as clues to its evolutionary origins. *Eur Arch Psychiat Clin Neurosci* 1995;**245**:61–9.

33. Done DJ, Johnstone EC, Frith CD, et al. Complications of pregnancy and delivery in relation to psychosis in adult life: data from the British perinatal mortality survey sample. *BMJ* 1991;**302**:1576–80.

34. Cannon TD, Kaprio J, Lonnqvist J, et al. The genetic epidemiology of schizophrenia in a Finnish twin cohort: a population-based modelling study. *Arch Gen Psychiat* 1998;**55**(1):67–74.

35. Jones P, Rodgers B, Murray R, et al. Child development risk factors for adult schizophrenia in the British 1946 birth cohort. *Lancet* 1994;**334**:1398–402.

36. Rantakallio P. Groups at risk in low birth weight infants and perinatal mortality. *Acta Paediat Scand Suppl* 1969;**193**:1–71.

37. Isohanni M, Jones PB, Moilanen K, et al. Early developmental milestones in adult schizophrenia and other psychoses. A 31-year follow-up of the North Finland 1966 birth cohort. *Schizophrenia Res* 2001;**52**:1–19.

38. Poulton R, Caspi A, Moffett TE, et al. Children's self reported psychotic symptoms and adult schizophreniform disorder: a 15 year longitudinal study. l. *Arch Gen Psychiat* 2000;**57**:1053–8.

39. Cannon M, Caspi A, Moffitt T, et al. Evidence for early, pan-developmental impairment specific to schizophreniform disorder. Results from a longitudinal birth cohort. *Arch Gen Psychiat* 2002;**59**(5):449–56.

40. Gervin M, Browne S, Lane A, et al. Spontaneous abnormal involuntary movements in first episode schizophrenia and schizophreniform disorder: baseline rate in a group of patients from an Irish catchment area. *Am J Psychiat* 1998;**155**:1202–6.

41. Ridler K, Veijola JM, Tanskanen P, et al. Fronto-cerebellar systems differentially associated with infant motor and adult executive functions in healthy adults compared to people with schizophrenia. *Arch Gen Psychiat*, submitted.

42. Ambelas A. Preschizophrenics: adding to the evidence, sharpening the focus. *Br J Psychiat* 1992;**160**:401–4.

43. Cannon-Spoor HE, Potkin SG, Wyatt RJ. Measurement of premorbid adjustment in chronic schizophrenia. *Schizophrenia Bull* 1982;**8**(3):470–84.

44. Foerster A, Lewis SW, Owen MJ, et al. Pre-morbid adjustment and personality in psychosis. Effects of sex and diagnosis. *Br J Psychiat* 1991;**158**:171–6.

45. Gittleman-Klein R, Klein DF. Premorbid and social adjustment and prognosis in schizophrenia. *J Psychiat Res* 1969;**7**:35–53.

46. Robins LN. *Deviant Children Grown Up. A Sociological and Psychiatric Study of Sociopathic Personality*. Baltimore: Williams & Wilkins, 1966.

47. Watt N, Lubensky A. Childhood roots of schizophrenia. *J Consult Clin Psychol* 1976;**44**:363–75.

48. Watt NF. Patterns of childhood social development in adult schizophrenics. *Arch Gen Psychiat* 1978;**35**:160–5.

49. Done DJ, Crow TJ, Johnstone EC, et al. Childhood antecedents of schizophrenia and affective illness: social adjustment at ages 7 and 11. *BMJ* 1994;**309**:699–703.

50. Jones P, Rodgers B, Murray R, et al. Childhood developmental risk factors for schizophrenia in the 1946 national birth cohort. *Lancet* 1994;**344**:1398–402.

51. Malmberg A, Lewis G, David A, Allebeck P. Premorbid adjustment and personality in people with schizophrenia. *Br J Psychiat* 1998;**172**:308–13.

52. Reichenberg A, Rabinowitz J, Weiser M, et al. Premorbid functioning in a national population of male twins discordant for psychoses. *Am J Psychiat* 2000; **157**:1514–6.

53. Rabinowitz J, Reichenberg A, Weiser M, et al. Cognitive and behavioural functioning in men with schizophrenia both before and shortly before first admission to hospital. Cross-sectional analyses. *Br J Psychiat* 2000;**177**:26–32.

54. Cannon TD, Rosso IM, Hollister JM, et al. A prospective cohort study of genetic and perinatal influences in the etiology of schizophrenia. *Schizophrenia Bull* 2000;**26**(2):351–66.

55. Aylward E, Walker E, Bettes B. Intelligence in schizophrenia: meta-analysis of the research. *Schizophrenia Bull* 1984;**10**:430–59.

56. Hunt JMcV, Cofer C. Psychological deficit. In: Hunt JMcV, editor. *Personality and the Behavior Disorders*. New York: Ronald Press, 1944.

57. Hunt H. A practical clinical test for organic brain damage. *J Appl Psychol* 1943;**27**:275–86.

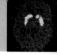

58. Lubin A, Gieseking CF, Williams HL. Direct measurement of cognitive deficit in schizophrenia. *J Consult Psychol* 1962;**26**:139–43.

59. Mason C. Pre-illness intelligence of mental hospital patients. *J Consult Psychol* 1956;**20**:297–300.

60. Rappoport SR, Webb WB. An attempt to study intellectual deterioration by pre-morbid testing. *J Consult Psychol* 1950;**14**:95–8.

61. Lane EA, Albee GW. Childhood intellectual development of adult schizophrenics. *J Abnorm Soc Psychol* 1963;**67**:186–9.

62. Albee GW, Lane EA, Corcoran C, et al. Childhood and inter-current intellectual performance of adult schizophrenics. *J Consult Psychol* 1963;**27**(4):364–6.

63. Russell AJ, Munro JC, Jones PB, et al. Schizophrenia and the myth of intellectual decline. *Am J Psychiat* 1997;**154**(5):635–9.

64. Pidgeon DA. Tests used in the 1954 and 1957 surveys. In: Douglas JWB, editor. *The Home and the School*. London: MacGibbon & Kee, 1964; pp. 129–32.

65. Pidgeon DA. Appendix: details of the fifteen year tests. In: Douglas JWB, Ross JM, Simpson HR, editors. *All Our Futures*. London: Peter Davies, 1968; pp. 194–7.

66. Jones PB. Childhood motor milestones and IQ prior to adult schizophrenia: results from a 43 year old British cohort. *Psychiatria Fennica* 1995;**26**:63–80.

67. David AS, Malmberg A, Brandt L, Allebeck P, Lewis G. IQ and risk for schizophrenia: a population-based cohort study. *Psychol Med* 1997;**27**(6):1311–23.

68. David AS, Cutting J. *The Neuropsychology of Schizophrenia*. Hove: Lawrence Erlbaum, 1994.

69. Cannon M, Jones P, Gilvarry K, et al. Premorbid social functioning in schizophrenia and bipolar disorder: similarities and differences. *Am J Psychiat* 1997;**154**(11):1544–50.

70. van Os J, Jones PB, Lewis GH, et al. Developmental precursors of affective illness in a general population birth cohort. *Arch Gen Psychiat* 1997;**54**:625–31.

71. Keith SJ, Regier DA, Rae DS. Schizophrenic disorders. In: Robins LN, Regier DA, editors. *Psychiatric Disorders in America: the Epidemiologic Catchment Area Study*. New York: Free Press, 1991; Chap. 3.

72. Kessler RC, McGonagle KA, Zhao S, et al. Lifetime and 12-month prevalence of DSM-III-R psychiatric disorders in the United States: results from the National Comorbidity Survey. *Arch Gen Psychiat* 1994;**52**:8–19.

73. Mason P, Wilkinson G. The prevalence of psychiatric morbidity. OPCS survey of psychiatric morbidity in Great Britain. *Br J Psychiat* 1996;**168**:1–3.

74. Office of Population Censuses and Surveys. *OPCS Surveys of Psychiatric Morbidity in Great Britain: Bulletin No. 1. The Prevalence of Psychiatric Morbidity Among Adults Aged 16–64 Living in Private Households in Great Britain*. London: OPCS.

75. Jablensky A, McGrath J, Herrman H, et al. *National Survey of Mental Health and Wellbeing. Report 4. People Living with Psychotic Illness: An Australian Study*. Australia: Commonwealth of Australia, 1999.

76. Torrey EF, Miller J. *The Invisible Plague. The Rise of Mental Illness from 1750 to the Present*. New Brunswick: Rutgers University Press, 2002; p. 416.

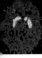
77. Der G, Gupta S, Murray RM. Is schizophrenia disappearing? *Lancet* 1990;**335**:513–6.

78. Eagles JM, Whalley LJ. Decline in the diagnosis of schizophrenia among first admissions to the Scottish mental hospitals from 1969–78. *Br J Psychiat* 1985;**146**:151–4.

79. Jones PB, Cannon M. Schizophrenia. In: Martyn CJ, Hughes RAC, editors. *The Epidemiology of Neurological Disorders*. London: BMJ Books, 1997.

80. Harrison G, Owens D, Holton A, et al. A prospective study of severe mental disorder in Afro-Caribbean patients. *Psychol Med* 1988;**18**:643–57.

81. Boydell J, van Os J, Lambri M, et al. Incidence of schizophrenia in south-east London between 1965 and 1997. *Br J Psychiat* 2003;**182**:45–9.

82. Allardyce J, Morrison G, McCreadie RG, et al. Schizophrenia is not disappearing in south-west Scotland. *Br J Psychiat* 2000;**177**:38–41.

83. Jablensky A, Sartorius N, Ernberg G, et al. Schizophrenia: manifestation, incidence and course in different cultures. A World Health Organisation ten country study. *Psychol Med* 1992; Monograph Suppl 20.

84. Mortensen PB, Penderson CB, Westergaard T, et al. Effects of family history and place and season of birth on the risk of schizophrenia. *New Engl J Med* 1999;**340**:603–8.

85. Pedersen CB, Mortensen PB. Family history, place and season of birth as risk factors for schizophrenia in Denmark: a replication and reanalysis. *Br J Psychiat* 2001;**179**:46–52.

86. Haukka J, Sivasaari J, Varilo T, et al. Regional variation in the incidence of schizophrenia in Finland: a study of birth cohort born from 1950 to 1969. *Psychol Med* 2001;**31**:1045–53.

87. Marcelis M, Takei N, van Os J. Urbanisation and risk for schizophrenia: does the effect operate before or around the time of illness onset? *Psychol Med* 1999;**29**(5):1197–203.

88. Lewis G, David A, Andreasson S, et al. Schizophrenia and city life. *Lancet* 1992;**340**:137–40.

89. Torrey EF, Bowler AE, Clark K. Urban birth and residence as risk factors for psychoses: an analysis of 1880 data. *Schizophrenia Res* 1997;**25**(3):169–76.

90. Faris R, Dunham HW. *Mental Disorders in Urban Areas*, 2nd ed. New York: Hafner Publishing, 1960.

91. Croudace TJ, Kayne R, Jones PB, et al. Non-linear relationship between an index of social deprivation, psychiatric admission prevalence and the incidence of psychosis. *Psychol Med* 2000;**30**:177–85.

92. van Os J, Castle DJ, Takei N, et al. Psychotic illness in ethnic minorities: clarification from the 1991 census. *Psychol Med* 1996;**26**(1):203–8.

93. King M, Coker E, Leavey G, et al. Incidence of psychotic illness in London: a comparison of ethnic groups. *BMJ* 1994;**309**:1115–9.

94. Thomas CS, Stone K, Osborn M, et al. Psychiatric morbidity and compulsory admission among UK-born Europeans, Afro-Caribbeans and Asians in Central Manchester 1993. *Br J Psychiat* 1993;**163**:91–9.

95. Wessley S, Castle D, Der G, et al. Schizophrenia and Afro-Caribbeans. A case-control study. *Br J Psychiat* 1991;**159**:795–801.

96. Selten JP, Sijben N. First admission rate for schizophrenia in immigrants to The Netherlands: the Dutch National Register. *Soc Psychiat Psychiat Epidemiol* 1994;**29**:71–2.

97. Burke AW. First admission rates and planning in Jamaica. *Soc Psychiat* 1974;**15**:17–9.

98. Hickling FW. Psychiatric hospital admission rates in Jamaica, 1971 and 1988. *Br J Psychiat* 1991;**159**:817–21.

99. Hollister M, Laing P, Mednick SA. Rhesus incompatibility as a risk factor for schizophrenia in male adults. *Arch Gen Psychiat* 1996;**53**:19–24.

100. McGovern D, Cope RV. First psychiatric admission rate of first and second generation Afro-Caribbeans. *Soc Psychiat* 1987;**22**:139–49.

101. Warner R. Time trends in schizophrenia: changes in obstetric risk factors with industrialization. *Schizophrenia Bull* 1995;**21**:483–500.

102. Khoury MJ, Beaty TH, Cohen BH. *Fundamentals of Genetic Epidemiology.* New York: OUP, 1993.

103. Khoury MJ, Beaty TH, Newill CA, et al. Genetic–environment interactions in chronic airways obstruction. *Am J Epidemiol* 1986;**15**:65–72.

104. Plomin R, DeFries J, McClearn GI, et al. *Behavioural Genetics.* New York: Freeman, 2001.

105. Gottesman IJ, Shields J. *Schizophrenia. The Epigenetic Puzzle.* Cambridge: Cambridge University Press, 1982; p. 258.

106. Kendler KS, Diehl SR. Schizophrenia: genetics. In: Kaplan HI, Sadock BJ, editors. *Comprehensive Textbook of Psychiatry VI*, Vol 1. Baltimore: Williams & Wilkins, 1995; pp. 942–57.

107. Kendler KS, McGuire M, Gruenberg AM, et al. The Roscommon family study. I. Methods, diagnosis of probands and risk of schizophrenia in relatives. *Arch Gen Psychiat* 1993;**50**:527–40.

108. Kendler KS, McGuire M, Gruenberg AM, et al. The Roscommon family study. II. The risk of nonschizophrenic, nonaffective psychosis in relatives. *Arch Gen Psychiat* 1993;**50**:645–52.

109. Kety SS, Wendler PH, Jacobson B, et al. Mental illness in the biological and adoptive relatives of schizophrenic adoptees. Replication of the Copenhagen study in the rest of Denmark. *Arch Gen Psychiat* 1994;**51**:442–55.

110. Kety SS. Mental illness in the biological and adoptive relatives of schizophrenic adoptees, findings relevant to genetic and environmental factors in etiology. *Am J Psychiat* 1983;**140**:720–7.

111. Tienari JP, Wynne CL, Laksy K, et al. Schizophrenics and their adopted-away offspring. The Finnish adoptive family study of schizophrenia. *Schizophrenia Res* 1997;**24**(1,2):43.

112. Tienari P. Interaction between genetic vulnerability and family environment: the Finnish adoptive study of schizophrenia. *Acta Psychiat Scand* 1991;**84**:460–5.

113. Gottesman II, Bertelsen A. Confirming unexpressed genotypes for schizophrenia. Risks in the offspring of Fischer's Danish identical and fraternal twins. *Arch Gen Psychiat* 1989;**46**:867–72.

114. Jones P, Murray R. The genetics of schizophrenia is the genetics of neurodevelopment. *Br J Psychiat* 1991;**158**:615–23.

115. Sham P. Genetic epidemiology. *Br Med Bull* 1996;**52**:408–33.

116. Parnas J, Cannon TD, Jacobsen B, et al. Lifetime DSM-III-R diagnostic outcomes in the offspring of schizophrenic mothers: results from the Copenhagen high-risk study. *Arch Gen Psychiat* 1993;**50**:707–14.

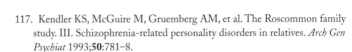

117. Kendler KS, McGuire M, Gruemberg AM, et al. The Roscommon family study. III. Schizophrenia-related personality disorders in relatives. *Arch Gen Psychiat* 1993;**50**:781–8.

118. Chapman JP, Chapman LJ, Kwapil TR. Scales for the assessment of schizotypy. In: Raine A, Lencz T, Mednick SA, editors. *Schizotypal Personality*. New York: Cambridge University Press, 1995; Chap. 5.

119. Kendler KS, McGuire M, Gruenberg AM, et al. Schizotypal symptoms and signs in the Roscommon family study: their factor structure and familial relationship with psychotic and affective disorder. *Arch Gen Psychiat* 1995;**52**:396–403.

120. Cannon TD, Zorrilla LE, Shtasel D, et al. Neuropsychological functioning in siblings discordant for schizophrenia and healthy volunteers. *Arch Gen Psychiat* 1994;**51**:89–102.

121. Kendler KS, McGuire M, Gruenberg AM, et al. The Roscommon family study. IV. Affective illness, anxiety disorders and alcoholism in relatives. *Arch Gen Psychiat* 1993;**50**:952–60.

122. Crow TJ. The continuum of psychosis and its genetic origins. The sixty-fifth Maudsley lecture. *Br J Psychiat* 1990;**156**:788–97.

123. Maier W, Lichterman D, Minges J, et al. Continuity and discontinuity of affective disorders and schizophrenia: results of a controlled family study. *Arch Gen Psychiat* 1993;**50**:871–83.

124. Squires-Wheeler E, Skodol AE, Bassett A, et al. DSM-III-R schizotypal personality traits in offspring of schizophrenic disorder, affective disorder, and normal control parents. *J Psychiat Res* 1989;**23**:229–39.

125. Kidd KK. Can we find genes for schizophrenia? *Am J Med Genet (Neuropsychiat Genet)* 1997;**74**:104–11.

126. Risch NJ. Linkage strategies for genetically-complex traits. I. Multilocus models. *Am J Hum Genet* 1990;**46**:222–8.

127. Kidd KK. Associations of disease with genetic markers. Deja vu all over again. *Am J Med Genet (Neuropsychiat Genet)* 1993;**48**:71–3.

128. Plomin R, Owen MJ, McGuffin P. The genetic basis of complex human behaviours. *Science* 1994;**264**:1733–9.

129. Harrison PJ, Weinberger DR. Schizophrenia genes, gene expression and neuropathology: on the matter of their convergence. *Molec Psychiat* 2005;**10**:40–68.

130. Claridge G. Schizotypy and schizophrenia. In: Bebbington P, McGuffin P, editors. *Schizophrenia: The Major Issues*. London: Heinemann, 1988; pp. 187–201.

131. Lewontin RC. The analysis of variance and the analysis of causes. *Am J Hum Genet* 1974;**26**:400–11.

132. Schizophrenia Linkage Collaborative Group for Chromosomes 3, 6 and 8. Additional support for schizophrenia linkage on chromosomes 6 and 8: a multicenter study. *Am J Med Genet (Neuropsychiat Genet)* 1996;**67**:580–94.

133. Straub RE, MacLean CJ, O'Neill FA, et al. A potential vulnerability locus for schizophrenia on chromosome 6p24-22: evidence for genetic heterogeneity. *Nat Genet* 1995;**11**:287–93.

134. Pulver AE, Lasseter VK, Kasch L, et al. Schizophrenia: a genome scan targets chromosomes 3p and 8p as potential sites of susceptibility genes. *Am J Hum Genet* 1995;**46**:222–8.

135. Peltonen L. All out for chromosome 6. *Nature* 1995;**378**:665–6.

136. Arolt V, Lencer R, Nolte A, et al. Eye tracking dysfunction is a putative phenotype susceptibility marker of schizophrenia and maps to a locus on chromosome 6p in families with multiple occurrence of the disease. *Am J Med Genet (Neuropsychiat Genet)* 1996;**67**:580–94.

137. Gill M, Vallada H, Collier D, et al. A combined analysis of D22S278 markers in affected sib-pairs: support for a susceptibility locus for schizophrenia at chromosome 22q12. *Am J Med Genet (Neuropsychiat Genet)* 1996;**67**:40–5.

138. Faraone S, Tsuang MT. Methods in psychiatric genetics. In: Tsuang MT, Tohen M, Zahner GEP, editors. *Textbook of Psychiatric Epidemiology.* New York: Wiley-Liss, 1995.

139. Owen M, McGuffin P. DNA and classical genetic markers in schizophrenia. *Eur Arch Psychiat Clin Neurosci* 1991;**240**:197–203.

140. Wright P, Donaldson PT, Underhill JA, et al. Genetic association of the HLA DRB1 gene locus on chromosome 6p21.3 with schizophrenia. *Am J Psychiat* 1996;**153**:1530–3.

141. Morrison PJ. Anticipating more anticipation. *Lancet* 1996;**347**:1132.

142. Gorwood P, Leboyer M, Falissard B, et al. Anticipation in schizophrenia: new light on a controversial problem. *Am J Psychiat* 1996;**153**:1173–7.

143. Petronis A, Kennedy JL. Unstable genes, unstable mind. *Am J Psychiat* 1995;**152**:164–72.

144. Kirov G, Murray R. The molecular genetics of schizophrenia: progress so far. *Molec Med Today* 1997;**March**:124–9.

145. O'Donovan MC, Guy C, Craddock N, et al. Expanded CAG repeats in schizophrenia and bipolar disorder. *Nature Genet* 1995;**10**:380–1.

146. Egan MF, Goldberg TE, Kolachana BS, et al. Effect of COMT Val108/158 Met genotype on frontal lobe function and risk for schizophrenia. *Proc Natl Acad Sci USA* 2001;**98**(12):6917–22.

147. Lachman HM, Papolos DF, Saito T, et al. Human catechol-O-methyltransferase pharmacogenetics: description of a functional polymorphism and its potential application to neuropsychiatric disorders. *Pharmacogenetics* 1996;**6**(3):243–50.

148. Gogos JA, Morgan M, Luine V, et al. Catechol-O-methyltransferase-deficient mice exhibit sexually dimorphic changes in catecholamine levels and behavior. *Proc Natl Acad Sci USA* 1998;**95**(17):9991–6.

149. Weinberger DR, Egan MF, Bertolino A, et al. Prefrontal neurons and the genetics of schizophrenia. *Biol Psychiat* 2001;**50**(11):825–44.

150. Glatt SJ, Faraone SV, Tsuang MT. Association between a functional catechol O-methyltransferase gene polymorphism and schizophrenia: meta-analysis of case-control and family-based studies. *Am J Psychiat* 2003;**160**(3):469–76.

151. Palmatier MA, Kang AM, Kidd KK. Global variation in the frequencies of functionally different catechol-O-methyltransferase alleles. *Biol Psychiat* 1999;**46**(4):557–67.

152. Goldberg TE, Egan MF, Gscheidle T, et al. Executive subprocesses in working memory: relationship to catechol-O-methyltransferase Val158Met genotype and schizophrenia. *Arch Gen Psychiat* 2003;**60**(9):889–96.

153. Gottesman II, Gould TD. The endophenotype concept in psychiatry. *Am J Psychiat* 2003;**160**:636–45.

154. Johnstone EC, Crow TJ, Frith CD, Husband J, Kreel L. Cerebral ventricular size and cognitive impairment in chronic schizophrenia. *Lancet* 1976;**2**:924–6.

155. Chua SE, McKenna PJ. Schizophrenia – a brain disease?: a critical review of structural and functional cerebral abnormality in the disorder. *Br J Psychiat* 1995;**166**:563–82.

156. Suddath RL, Christison GW, Torrey EF, et al. Anatomical abnormalities in the brains of monozygotic twins discordant for schizophrenia. *New Engl J Med* 1990;**322**:789–94.

157. Wright IC, Rabe-Hesketh S, Woodruff PW, David AS, Murray RM, Bullmore ET. Meta-analysis of regional brain volumes in schizophrenia. *Am J Psychiat* 2000;**157**(1):16–25.

158. Winterer G, Coppola R, Egan MF, et al. Functional and effective frontotemporal connectivity and genetic risk for schizophrenia. *Biol Psychiat* 2003;**54**(11):1181–92.

159. Meyer-Lindenberg A, Poline JB, Kohn PD, et al. Evidence for abnormal cortical functional connectivity during working memory in schizophrenia. *Am J Psychiat* 2001;**158**(11):1809–17.

160. Harrison PJ, Weinberger DR. Schizophrenia genes, gene expression, and neuropathology: on the matter of their convergence. *Molec Psychiat* 2005;**10**(1):40–68.

161. Mimmack ML, Ryan M, Baba H, et al. Gene expression analysis in schizophrenia: reproducible upregulation of several members of the apolipoprotein L family located in a high susceptibility locus for schizophrenia on chromosome 22. *Proc Natl Acad Sci USA* 2002;**99**(7):4680–5.

162. Geddes JR, Lawrie SM. Obstetric complications and schizophrenia: a meta-analysis. *Br J Psychiat* 1995;**167**:786–93.

163. Lewis SW, Owen MJ, Murray RM. Obstetric complications and schizophrenia: methodology and mechanisms. In: Schultz SC, Tamminga CA, editors. *Schizophrenia: A Scientific Focus*. New York: Oxford University Press, 1989; pp. 56–9.

164. Buka S, Tsuang MT, Lipsitt LP. Pregnancy-delivery complications and psychiatric diagnosis: a prospective study. *Arch Gen Psychiat* 1993;**50**:151–6.

165. Jones P, Rantakallio P, Hartikainen A-L, et al. Schizophrenia as a long-term outcome of pregnancy, delivery and perinatal complications: a 28-year follow-up of the 1966 North Finland general population birth cohort. *Am J Psychiat* 1998;**155**(3):355–64.

166. Kendell RE, Juszczak E, Cole SK. Obstetric complications and schizophrenia: a case-control study based on standardised obstetric records. *Br J Psychiat* 1996;**168**:556–61.

167. Mednick SA, Machon RA, Huttunen MO, et al. Adult schizophrenia following prenatal exposure to an influenza epidemic. *Arch Gen Psychiat* 1988;**45**:171–6.

168. O'Callaghan E, Sham P, Takei N, et al. Schizophrenia after prenatal exposure to the 1957 A2 influenza epidemic. *Lancet* 1991;**337**:1248–50.

169. Sham PC, O'Callaghan E, Takei N, et al. Increased risk of schizophrenia following prenatal exposure to influenza. *Br J Psychiat* 1992;**160**:461–6.

170. Susser E, Lin P. Schizophrenia after prenatal exposure to the Dutch hunger winter of 1944–1945. *Arch Gen Psychiat* 1992;**49**:983–8.

171. Susser E, Neugebauer R, Hoek HW, et al. Schizophrenia after prenatal famine: further evidence. *Arch Gen Psychiat* 1996;**53**:25–31.

172. Huttunen MO, Niskanen P. Prenatal loss of father and psychiatric disorders. *Arch Gen Psychiat* 1978;**35**:429–31.

173. Myhrman A, Rantakallio P, Isohanni M, et al. Does unwantedness of a pregnancy predict schizophrenia? *Br J Psychiat* 1996;**169**:637–40.

174. Rantakallio P, Jones P, Moring J, et al. Association between central nervous system infections during childhood and adult onset schizophrenia and other psychoses: a 28-year follow-up. *Int J Epidemiol* 1997;**26**(4):837–43.

175. Buka SL, Tsuang MT, Torrey EF, et al. Maternal cytokine levels during pregnancy and adult psychosis. *Brain Behav Immun* 2001;**15**(4):411–20.

176. Buka SL, Tsuang MT, Torrey EF, et al. Maternal infections and subsequent psychosis among offspring. *Arch Gen Psychiat* 2001;**58**(11):1032–7.

177. McGrath JJ, Murray RM. Risk factors for schizophrenia – from conception to birth. In: Hirsch S, Weinberger D, editors. *Schizophrenia*. Oxford: Blackwell, 1995; pp. 187–205.

178. Bracha HS, Torrey EF, Gottesman II, et al. Second-trimester markers of fetal size in schizophrenia: a study of monozygotic twins. *Am J Psychiat* 1992;**149**:1355–61.

179. Davis JO, Bracha HS. Prenatal growth markers in schizophrenia: a monozygotic co-twin control study. *Am J Psychiat* 1996;**153**:1166–72.

180. Bradbury TN, Miller GA. Season of birth in schizophrenia: a review of the evidence, methodology and etiology. *Psychol Bull* 1985;**98**:569–94.

181. Cotter D, Larkin C, Waddington JL, et al. Season of birth in schizophrenia: clue or cul-de-sac? In: Waddington JL, Buckley PB, editors. *The Neurodevelopmental Basis of Schizophrenia*. RG Landes, 1995.

182. Andreasson S, Allebeck P, Engström A, et al. Cannabis and schizophrenia. *Lancet* 1987;**2**:1483–6.

183. Arseneault L, Cannon M, Poulton R, et al. Cannabis use in adolescence and risk for adult psychosis: longitudinal prospective study. *BMJ* 2002;**325**:1212–3.

184. Fergusson DM, Horwood LJ, Swain-Campbell NR. Cannabis dependence and psychotic symptoms in young people. *Psychol Med* 2003;**33**:15–21.

185. Zammit S, Allebeck P, Andreasson S, et al. Self reported cannabis use as a risk factor for schizophrenia in Swedish conscripts of 1969: historical cohort study. *BMJ* 2002;**325**:1199.

186. van Os J, Bak M, Bijl RV, et al. Cannabis use and psychosis: a longitudinal population-based study. *Am J Epidemiol* 2002;**156**:319–27.

187. Arseneault L, Cannon M, Witton J, Murray RM. Causal association between cannabis and psychosis: examination of the evidence. *Br J Psychiat* 2004;**184**:110–7.

188. Roiser JP, Cook LJ, Cooper JD, et al. Association of a functional polymorphism in the serotonin transporter gene with abnormal emotional processing in ecstasy users. *Am J Psychiat* 2005;**162**(3):609–12.

189. McGorry P, Yung AR, Philips LJ. The "close in" or ultra high risk model: a safe and effective strategy for research and clinical intervention in prepsychotic mental disorder. *Schizophrenia Bull* 2003;**29**:771–90.

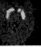
190. Nasmiranhim M, Buckley PF. The prodrome of schizophrenia. *Curr Psychiat* 2005;**18**(2):195–221.

191. Johnstone EC, Lawrie SM, Cosway R. What does the Edinburgh high risk study tell us about schizophrenia? *Am J Med Genet* 2002;**114**:906–12.

192. McGlashan TH, Miller TJ, Woods SW. Pre-onset detection and intervention research in schizophrenia psychoses: current estimates of benefit and risks. *Schizophrenia Bull* 2001;**27**:563–70.

193. Tsuang NT, Storm WS, Sieddman LJ, et al. Treatment of nonpsychotic relatives of patients with schizophrenia: 4 case studies. *Biol Psychiat* 1999;**45**:1412–8.

194. McGorry PD, Yung AR, Philips LJ, et al. Randomized, controlled trial of interventions designed to reduce the risk of progression to first episode psychosis in a clinical sample with subthreshold symptoms. *Arch Gen Psychiat* 2002;**59**:921–8.

195. Stahl SM. Prophylactic antipsychotics: do they keep you from catching schizophrenia? *J Clin Psychiat* 2004;**65**:1445–6.

196. Lewis SW. The secondary schizophrenias. In: Hirsch SR, Weinberger DR, editors. *Schizophrenia*. Cambridge: Blackwell Science, 1995; pp. 324–40.

197. Ron M, Harvey I. The brain in schizophrenia. *J Neurol Neurosurg Psychiat* 1990;**53**:725–6.

198. Guze SB. Biological psychiatry: is there any other kind? *Psychol Med* 1989;**19**:315–23.

199. Bynum WF. Psychiatry in its historical context. In: Shepherd M, Zangwill OL, editors. *Handbook of Psychiatry*, Vol. 1. Cambridge: CUP General Psychopathology, 1983; pp. 12–3.

200. Murray RM. Neurodevelopmental schizophrenia: the rediscovery of dementia praecox. *Br J Psychiat* 1994;**165**(Suppl 25):6–12.

201. Kraepelin E. Dementia praecox and paraphrenia. Translated by Barclay RM from: Robertson G, editor. *Text Book of Psychiatry*, Vol. iii, Part ii, section on Endogenous Dementias, 8th ed. Edinburgh: Livingstone, 1919.

202. Pick A. *Über Primäre Demenz*. Wandervorträge, 1891.

203. Diem O. Die einfach demente Form de Dementia praecox. *Arch Psychiat* 1903;**37**:111–87.

204. Pinel Ph. *Traité Médico-philosophique sur l'Aliénation Mentale*. Paris: R. Caille, Ravier, 1801.

205. Morel BA. *Etudes Cliniques: Traité Théorique et Pratique des Maladies Mentales*. Paris: Masson, 1852.

206. Morel BA. *Traité des Maladies Mentales*. Paris: Masson, 1860.

207. Snell L. Uber Monomanie als primäre Form der Seelenstörung. *Allg Z Psychiat* 1865;**22**:368–81.

208. Kahlbaum KL. *Die Katatonie oder das Spannungsirresein*. Berlin: Hirschwald, 1874.

209. Hecker E. Die Hebephrenie. *Virchows Arch Pathol Anat* 1871;**52**:394–429.

210. Fink E. Beitrag zur Kenntnis des Jugendirreseins. *Allg Z Psychiat* 1881;**37**:490–520.

211. Murray RM. Schizophrenia. In: Hill P, Murray RM, Thorley A, editors. *Essentials of Postgraduate Psychiatry*. Cambridge: CUP, 1986; pp. 339–79.

212. Minkowski E. Le trouble essential de la schizophrenie et al., pensee schiz-ophrenique. *La Schizophrenie*, Chap. 2. Paris: Payot, 1927. Translated in: Cutting J, Shepherd M. *The Clinical Roots of the Schizophrenia Concept.* Cambridge: CUP, 1987; pp. 189–212.

213. Stransky E. Towards an understanding of certain symptoms of dementia praecox. Zur Auffassung gewisser Symptome der Dementia Praecox. *Neurol Centralblatt* 1904;**23**:1137–43. Translated in: Cutting J, Shepherd M. *The Clinical Roots of the Schizophrenia Concept.* Cambridge: CUP, 1987; pp. 36–41.

214. Castle DJ, Murray RM. The neurodevelopmental basis of sex differences in schizophrenia. *Psychol Med* 1991;**21**:565–75.

215. Schneider K. *Clinical Psychopathology.* Translated by Hamilton MW. New York: Grune & Stratton, 1959.

216. Cooper JE, Kendell RE, Gurland BJ, et al. *Psychiatric Diagnosis in New York and London.* Oxford: Oxford University Press, 1972.

217. Jackson JH. *Selected Writings of JH Jackson.* London: Hodder & Stoughton, 1931.

218. Crow TJ. Positive and negative symptoms of schizophrenia and the role of dopamine. *Br J Psychiat* 1980;**137**:383–6.

219. Andreasen NC. *Can Schizophrenia be Localised in the Brain?* Washington, DC: American Psychiatric Press, 1986.

220. Carpenter WT Jr, Heinrichs WD, Alphs LD. Treatment of negative symptoms. *Schizophrenia Bull* 1985;**11**:440–52.

221. Braff DL. Information processing and attention dysfunctions in schizo-phrenia. *Schizophrenia Bull* 1993;**19**:233–59.

222. Mesulam MD, Geschwind N. On the possible role of the limbic cortex and its limbic connections in the process of attention in schizophrenia. *J Psychiat Res* 1983;**14**:249–61.

223. Ingvar DH, Franzen G. Abnormalities of cerebral blood flow distribution in patients with chronic schizophrenia. *Acta Psychiat Scand* 1974;**50**:425–62.

224. Liddle PF, Friston KJ, Herold S, et al. A PET study of word generation in schizophrenia. *Schizophrenia Res* 1994;**11**:168.

225. Wernike C. *Grundrisse der Psychiatrie.* Leipzig: Thieme, 1906.

226. Jones PB. The early origins of schizophrenia. *Br Med Bull* 1997;**53**(1):135–55.

227. Lewis SW. Congenital risk factors for schizophrenia. *Psychol Med* 1989;**19**:5–13.

228. Murray RM, Jones PB, O'Callaghan E, et al. Genes, viruses and neurode-velopmental schizophrenia. *J Psychiat Res* 1992;**26**(4):225–35.

229. Kostovic I, Rakic P. Developmental history of the transient subplate zone in the visual and somatosensory cortex of the macaque monkey and human brain. *J Comp Neurol* 1990;**297**(3):441–70.

230. McGuire PK, Frith CD. Disordered functional connectivity in schizo-phrenia. *Psychol Med* 1996;**26**:663–7.

231. Friston KJ. Dysfunctional connectivity in schizophrenia. *World Psychiat* 2002;**1**(2):66–71.

232. Hirsch SR, Shepherd M. *Themes and Variations in European Psychiatry.* Bristol: John Wright, 1974.

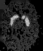
233. Kendler KS, Gallagher TJ, Abelson JM, et al. Lifetime prevalence, demographic risk factors, and diagnostic validity of nonaffective psychosis as assessed in a US community sample. The National Comorbidity Survey. *Arch Gen Psychiat* 1996;**53**:1022–31.

234. Lehman AF. Developing an outcomes-oriented approach for the treatment of schizophrenia. *J Clin Psychiat* 1999;**60**:30–5.

235. Emsley R, Oosthuizen P. Evidence-based pharmacotherapy of schizophrenia. *Int J Neuropsychopharmacol* 2004;**7**(2):219–38.

236. Sartorius N, Fleischhacker WW, Gjerris A, et al. The usefulness and uses of second generation antipsychotic medications. *Curr Opin Psychiat* 2002;**15**(monograph):S1–51.

237. Waddington JL, O'Callaghan E. What makes an antipsychotic 'atypical'? Conserving the definition. *CNS Drugs* 1997;**7**:341–6.

238. Glazer WM. Extrapyramidal side effects, tardive dyskinesia, and the concept of schizophrenia. *J Clin Psychiat* 2000;**61**:16–21.

239. Ellenbroek BA. Treatment of schizophrenia. A preclinical and clinical evaluation of neuroleptic drugs. *Pharmacol Ther* 1993;**57**:1–78.

240. Creese I, Burt DR, Snyder S. Dopamine receptor binding predicts clinical and pharmacological properties of antischizophrenic drugs. *Science* 1976;**192**:481–3.

241. Kapur S, Remmington G. Dopamine D2 receptors and their role in atypical antipsychotic action: still necessary and maybe even sufficient. *Biol Psychiat* 2001;**50**:873–83.

242. Kapur S, Zipursky R, Remmington G, et al. Relationship between dopamine D2 occupancy, clinical response, and side effects: a double blind PET study of first episode schizophrenia. *Am J Psychiat* 2000;**157**:514–20.

243. Kapur S, Zipursky R, Remmington G, et al. Clinical and therapeutic implications of 5HT2 and D2 receptor occupancy of clozapine, risperidone, and olanzapine in schizophrenia. *Am J Psychiat* 1999;**156**:286–93.

244. Kapur S, Zipursky R, Remmington G, et al. PET evidence that loxapine is an equipotent blocker of 5HT2 and receptors: implications for the treatment of schizophrenia. *Am J Psychiat* 1997;**154**:1525–9.

245. Xiberas X, Martinot JL, Mallet L, et al. Extrastriatal and striatal D2 dopamine receptor with haloperidol or new antipsychotic drugs in patients with schizophrenia. *Br J Psychiat* 2001;**179**:503–8.

246. Allen MH. Managing the agitated psychotic patient: a reappraisal of the evidence. *J Clin Psychiat* 2000;**61**:11–20.

247. Gilbert P, Harris MJ, McAdams LA, et al. Neuroleptic withdrawal in schizophrenic patients: a review of the literature. *Arch Gen Psychiat* 1995;**52**:173–88.

248. Adams CE, Fenton M, David AS. Systematic meta-review of depot antipsychotic drugs for people with schizophrenia. *Br J Psychiat* 2001;**179**:290–9.

249. Conley RR, Kelly DL. Management of treatment resistance in schizophrenia. *Biol Psychiat* 2001;**50**:898–911.

250. Keefe RSE, Silva SG, Perkins DO, et al. The effects of atypical antipsychotic drugs on neurocognitive impairment in schizophrenia: a review and meta-analysis. *Schizophrenia Bull* 1999;**25**(2):201–22.

251. Harvey PD, Keefe RSE. Studies of cognitive change in patients with schizophrenia following treatment with atypical antipsychotics. *Am J Psychiat* 2001;**158**:176–84.

252. Cunningham-Owens DG. *A Guide to the Extrapyramidal Side Effects of Antipsychotic Drugs*. Cambridge: Cambridge University Press, 1999.

253. Kane JM. Tardive dyskinesia: epidemiological and clinical presentation. In: Bloom FE, Kupfer DJ, editors. *Psychopharmacology, A Fourth Generation of Progress*. New York: Raven Press, 1995; pp. 1485–95.

254. Glazer WM. Expected incidence of tardive dyskinesia associated with typical antipsychotics. *J Clin Psychiat* 2000;**61**:15–20.

255. Correll CU, Leucht S, Kane JM. Lower risk for tardive dyskinesia associated with second-generation antipsychotics: a systematic review of 1-year studies. *Am J Psychiat* 2004;**161**(3):414–25.

256. Buckley PF, Adityanjee, Sajatovic M. Neuroleptic malignant syndrome. In: Bashir Y, et al., editors. *Textbook of Neuromuscular Disorders*. Philadelphia: Butterworth-Heinemann, 2001.

257. Glazer WM, Kane JM. Depot neuroleptics therapy: an underutilized treatment option. *J Clin Psychiat* 1992;**53**:426–30.

258. Arana GW. An overview of side effects caused by typical antipsychotics. *J Clin Psychiat* 2000;**61**:5–11.

259. Percudani M, Barbui C, Tansella M. Effect of second-generation antipsychotics on employment and productivity in individuals with schizophrenia: an economic perspective. *Pharmacoeconomics* 2004;**22**(11):701–18.

260. Frangou S, Lewis M. Atypical antipsychotics in ordinary clinical practice: a pharmacoepidemiologic survey in a south London service. *Eur Psychiat* 2000;**15**:200–26.

261. Geddes J, Freemantle N, Harrison P, et al. Atypical antipsychotics in the treatment of schizophrenia: systematic overview and regression analysis. *BMJ* 2000;**321**:1371–6.

262. Rosenheck R, Perlick D, Bingham S, et al. Effectiveness and cost of olanzapine and haloperidol in the treatment of schizophrenia: a randomized controlled trial. *JAMA* 2003;**290**(20):2693–702.

263. Davis J, Chen N, Glick ID. A metanalysis of the efficacy of second-generation antipsychotics. *Arch Gen Psychiat* 2003;**60**(6):553–64.

264. Lehman AF, Lieberman JA, Dixon LB, et al. American Psychiatric Association, Steering Committee on Practice Guidelines. Practice guidelines for the treatment of patients with schizophrenia, second edition. *Am J Psychiat* 2004;**161**(2, Suppl):1–56.

265. Lehman AF, Kreyenbuhl J, Buchanan RW, et al. The Schizophrenia Patient Outcomes Research Team (PORT): updated treatment recommendations 2003. *Schizophrenia Bull* 2004;**30**(2):193–217.

266. Miller AL, Hall CS, Buchanan RW, et al. The Texas Medication Algorithm Project antipsychotic algorithm for schizophrenia: 2003 update. *J Clin Psychiat* 2004;**65**(4):500–8.

267. Leucht S, Barnes TR, Kissling W, et al. Relapse prevention in schizophrenia with new-generation antipsychotics: a systematic review of exploratory meta-analysis of randomized, controlled trials. *Am J Psychiat* 2003;**160**(7):1209–22.

268. Richelson E, Souder T. Binding of antipsychotic drugs to human brain receptors – focus on new generation compounds. *Life Sci* 2000;**68**:29–39.

269. Kane J, Honigfeld G, Singer J, et al. The Clozapine Collaborative Group. Clozapine for the treatment-resistant schizophrenic: a double-blind comparison with chlorpromazine. *Arch Gen Psychiat* 1988;**45**:789–96.

270. Rosenheck R, Cramer J, Xu W, et al. Department of Veterans Affairs Cooperative Study Group of Clozapine in Refractory Schizophrenia. A comparison of clozapine and haloperidol in hospitalized patients with refractory schizophrenia. *New Engl J Med* 1997;**337**:809–15.

271. Wallbeck K, Cheine M, Essali A, Adam C. Evidence for clozapine's effectiveness in schizophrenia: a systematic review and metanalysis of randomized trials. *Am J Psychiat* 1999;**156**:990–9.

272. Chakos M, Lieberman J, Hoffman E. Effectiveness of second-generation antipsychotics in patients with treatment-resistant schizophrenia: a review and meta-analysis of randomized trials. *Am J Psychiat* 2001;**158**:518–26.

273. Casey DE. Effects of clozapine therapy in schizophrenic individuals at risk for tardive dyskinesia. *J Clin Psychiat* 1998;**59**(3, Suppl):31–7.

274. Rosenheck R, Dunn L, Peszke M, et al. Department of Veterans Affairs Cooperative Study Group on Clozapine in Refractory Schizophrenia. Impact of clozapine on negative symptoms and on the deficit syndrome in refractory schizophrenia. *Am J Psychiat* 1999;**156**:88–93.

275. Walker AM, Lanza L, Arelliano F, et al. Mortality in current and former users of clozapine. *Epidemiology* 1997;**6**:671–7.

276. Meltzer HY, Alphs L, Green AI, et al. Clozapine treatment for suicidality in schizophrenia. International Suicide Prevention Trial (InterSePT). *Arch Gen Psychiat* 2003;**60**:82–91.

277. Glazer WM, Dickson RA. Clozapine reduces violence and persistent aggression in schizophrenia. *J Clin Psychiat* 1998;**59**:8–14.

278. Buckley PF. Substance abuse and schizophrenia: a review. *J Clin Psychiat* 1998;**59**:26–30.

279. Keefe R, Silva S, Perkins D, et al. The effects of atypical antipsychotic drugs on neurocognitive impairment in schizophrenia: a review and meta-analysis. *Schizophrenia Bull* 1999;**25**:201–22.

280. Conley RR. Optimizing treatment with clozapine. *J Clin Psychiat* 1998;**59**(3, Suppl):44–9.

281. Honigfeld G, Arellano F, Sethi J, et al. Reducing clozapine-related morbidity and mortality: five years of experience with the Clozaril National Registry. *J Clin Psychiat* 1998;**59**(3, Suppl):3–7.

282. Kilian J, Kerr K, Lawrence C, et al. Myocarditis and cardiomyopathy associated with clozapine. *Lancet* 1999;**354**:1841–5.

283. Coodin S, Ballegeer T. Clozapine therapy and pulmonary embolism. *Can J Psychiat* 2000;**45**:395.

284. Allison DB, Mentore JL, Moonseong H, et al. Antipsychotic-induced weight gain: a comprehensive research synthesis. *Am J Psychiat* 1999;**156**:1686–96.

285. American Diabetes Association, American Psychiatric Association, American Association of Clinical Endocrinologists, North American Association for the Study of Obesity. Consensus Development Conference on Antipsychotic Drugs and Obesity and Diabetes. *Diabetes Care* 2004;**27**:596–601.

286. Casey DE, Haupt DW, Newcomer JW, et al. Antipsychotic-induced weight gain and metabolic abnormalities: implications for increased mortality in patients with schizophrenia. *J Clin Psychiat* 2004;**65**(Suppl 7):4–18.

287. Marder SR, Essock SM, Miller AL, et al. Physical health monitoring of patients with schizophrenia. *Am J Psychiat* 2004;**161**:1334–49.

288. Baptista T, Zarate J, Joober R, et al. Drug induced weight gain, an impediment to successful pharmacotherapy: focus on antipsychotics. *Curr Drug Targets* 2004;**5**(3):279–99.

289. Meyer JM, Koro CE. The effects of antipsychotic therapy on serum lipids: a comprehensive review. *Schizophrenia Res* 2004;**70**(1):1–17.

290. Henderson DC, Cagliero E, Gray C, et al. Clozapine, diabetes mellitus, and weight gain, and lipid abnormalities: a five year naturalistic study. *Am J Psychiat* 2000;**157**:975–81.

291. Citrome LL. The increase in risk of diabetes mellitus from exposure to second-generation antipsychotic agents. *Drugs Today* 2004;**40**(5):445–64.

292. Marder SR, Fleishacker WF. Risperidone and olanzapine: experience in clinical practice. In: Buckley PF, Waddington JL, editors. *Schizophrenia and Mood Disorders: The New Drug Therapies in Clinical Practice*. Bristol: Butterworth-Heinemann, 2000.

293. Keck PE, Wilson DR, Strakowski SM, et al. Clinical predictors of acute risperidone response in schizophrenia, schizoaffective disorder and psychotic mood disorders. *J Clin Psychiat* 1995;**56**:466–70.

294. Reveley MA, Libretto SE. RIS-GBR-31 investigators. Treatment outcomes in patients with chronic schizophrenia during long-term administration with risperidone. *J Clin Psychopharmacol* 2004;**24**(3):260–7.

295. Vieta E, Goikolee JM. Atypical antipsychotics: new options for mania and maintenance therapy. *Bipolar Disorder* 2005;**7**(Suppl 4):21–33.

296. Green MF, Marshall BD, Wirshing W, et al. Does risperidone improve verbal working memory in treatment-resistant schizophrenia? *Am J Psychiat* 1997;**154**:799–804.

297. Chengappa KNR, Sheth S, Brar JS, et al. A clinical audit of the first 142 patients who received risperidone at a state psychiatric hospital. *J Clin Psychiat* 1999;**60**:373–8.

298. Currier GW, Chou JC, Feifel D, et al. Acute treatment of psychotic agitation: a randomized comparison of oral treatment with risperidone and lorazepam versus intramuscular treatment with haloperidol and lorazepam. *J Clin Psychiat* 2004;**65**(3):386–94.

299. Kane JM, Eerdekens M, Lindenmayer JP, et al. Long-acting injectable risperidone: efficacy and safety of the first long-acting atypical antipsychotic. *Am J Psychiat* 2003;**160**:1125–32.

300. Fleischhacker WW, Eedekens M, Karcher K. Treatment of schizophrenia with long-acting injectable risperidone: a 12-month open-label trial of the first long-acting second generation antipsychotic. *J Clin Psychiat* 2003;**64**:1250–7.

301. Emsley RA. Risperidone in the treatment of first-episode psychotic patients: a double-blind multicenter study. *Schizophrenia Bull* 1999;**25**:721–9.

302. Csernansky JG, Mahmoud R, Brenner R, et al. The Risperidone User 79 Study Group. A comparison of risperidone and haloperidol for the prevention of relapse in patients with schizophrenia. *New Engl J Med* 2002;**346**:16–22.

303. Koro CE, Fedder DO, L'Italien GJ, et al. Assessment of independent effect of olanzapine and risperidone on risk of diabetes among patients with schizophrenia: population based nested case-control study. *BMJ* 2002;**325**(7358):243.

304. Bronson B, Lindenmeyer JP. Adverse effects of high-dose olanzapine in treatment-refractory schizophrenia. *J Clin Psychopharmacol* 2000;**20**:382–4.

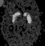

305. Tollefson GD, Beasley CM, Tran PV, et al. Olanzapine versus haloperidol in the treatment of schizophrenia and schizoaffective and schizophreniform disorders: results of an international collaborative trial. *Am J Psychiat* 1997;**154**:457–65.

306. Tollefson GD, Sanger TM. Negative symptoms: a path analytic approach to a double-blind, placebo- and haloperidol-controlled clinical trial with olanzapine. *Am J Psychiat* 1997;**154**:466–74.

307. Tollefson GD, Sanger TM, Lu Y, et al. Depressive signs and symptoms in schizophrenia: a prospective blinded trial of olanzapine and haloperidol. *Arch Gen Psychiat* 1998;**55**:250–8.

308. Purdon S, Jones B, Stip E. Neuropsychological change in early phase schizophrenia during 12 months of treatment with olanzapine, risperidone, or haloperidol. *Arch Gen Psychiat* 2000;**57**:249–58.

309. Wright P, Birkett M, David SR, et al. A double blind placebo controlled comparison of intramuscular olanzapine and intramuscular haloperidol in the treatment of acute agitation in schizophrenia. *Am J Psychiat* 2001;**158**:1149–51.

310. Conley RR, Kelly DL, Gale EA. Olanzapine response in treatment refractory patients with a history of substance abuse. *Schizophrenia Res* 1998;**33**:95–101.

311. Sanger TM, Lieberman JA, Tohen M, et al. Olanzapine versus haloperidol treatment in first-episode psychosis. *Am J Psychiat* 1999;**156**:79–87.

312. Lieberman JA, Tollefson G, Tohen M, et al. HGDH Study Group. Comparative efficacy and safety of atypical and conventional antipsychotic drugs in first-episode psychosis: a randomized, double-blind trial of olanzapine versus haloperidol. *Am J Psychiat* 2003;**160**(8):1396–404.

313. Tran PV, Dellva MA, Tollefson G, et al. Oral olanzapine vs oral haloperidol in the maintenance treatment of schizophrenia and related psychoses. *Br J Psychiat* 1998;**172**:499–505.

314. Lindenmayer JP. Treatment refractory schizophrenia. *Psychiat Quart* 2000;**71**:373–84.

315. Conley RR, Tamminga CA, Bartko JJ, et al. Olanzapine compared with chlorpromazine in treatment-resistant schizophrenia. *Am J Psychiat* 1998;**155**:914–20.

316. Bitter I, Dossenbach MR, Brook S, et al. Olanzapine HGCK Study Group. Olanzapine versus clozapine in treatment-resistant or treatment-intolerant schizophrenia. *Prog Neuropsychopharmacol Biol Psychiat* 2004;**28**(1):173–80.

317. Volavka J, Czobor P, Sheitman B, et al. Clozapine, olanzapine, risperidone, and haloperidol in the treatment of patients with chronic schizophrenia and schizoaffective disorder. *Am J Psychiat* 2002;**159**:255–62.

318. Tollefson GD, Beasley CM, Tamura RN, et al. Blind, controlled, long-term study of the comparative incidence of treatment-emergent tardive dyskinesia with olanzapine or haloperidol. *Am J Psychiat* 1997;**154**:1248–54.

319. Kinon BJ, Jeste DV, Kollack-Walker S, et al. Olanzapine treatment for tardive dyskinesia in schizophrenia patients: a prospective clinical trial with patients randomized to blinded dose reduction periods. *Prog Neuropsychopharmacol Biol Psychiat* 2004;**6**:985–96.

320. Melkersson K, Hutling A, Brismar K. Elevated levels of insulin, leptin, and blood lipids in olanzapine-treated patients with schizophrenia or related psychoses. *J Clin Psychiat* 2000;**61**:742–9.

321. Sacchetti E, Guarneri L, Bravi D. H antagonist nizatidine may control olanzapine-associated weight gain in schizophrenic patients. *Biol Psychiat* 2000;**48**:167–8.

322. Goldstein JM. Quetiapine fumarate (seroquel): a new atypical antipsychotic. *Drugs Today* 1999;**35**(3):193–210.

323. Kapur S, Zipursky RB, Jones C, et al. A positron emission tomography study of quetiapine in schizophrenia: a preliminary finding of an antipsychotic effect with only transiently high dopamine D2 receptor occupancy. *Arch Gen Psychiat* 2000;**57**:553–9.

324. Arvantis LA, Miller BG. Seroquel Trial 12 Study Group. Multiple fixed doses of "Seroquel" (quetiapine) in patients with acute exacerbation of schizophrenia: a comparison with haloperidol and placebo. *Biol Psychiat* 1997;**42**:233–46.

325. Emsley RA, Raniwalla J, Bailey PJ. On behalf of the PRIZE Study Group. A comparison of the effects of quetiapine (Seroquel) and haloperidol in schizophrenic patients with a history of and a demonstrated partial response to conventional antipsychotic treatment. *Int Clin Psychopharmacol* 2000;**15**:121–31.

326. Mullen J, Jibson MD, Sweitzer D. A comparison of the relative safety, efficacy and tolerability of quetiapine and risperidone in outpatients with schizophrenia and other psychotic disorders: the QUEST study. *Clin Ther* 2001;**23**:1839–54.

327. Velligan DI, Newcomer J, Peltz J, et al. Does cognitive function improve with quetiapine in comparison with haloperidol. *Schizophrenia Res* 2002;**53**:239–48.

328. Hellewell JSE, Centillon M, Amermeron Hands D. Seroquel: evidence for efficacy in the treatment of hostility and aggression. *Schizophrenia Res* 1998;**29**:154–5.

329. Good KP, Kiss I, Buiteman C, et al. Improvement in cognitive functioning in patients with first-episode psychosis during treatment with quetiapine: an interim analysis. *Br J Psychiat* 2002;**43**(Suppl):s45–9.

330. Buckley PF. Maintenance treatment of schizophrenia with quetiapine. *Human Psychopharmacol* 2004;**19**:121–4.

331. Buckley PF, Goldstein JM, Emsley RA. Efficacy and tolerability of quetiapine in poorly responsive, chronic schizophrenia. *Schizophrenia Res* 2004;**66**(2–3):143–50.

332. Pierre JM, Wirshing DA, Wirshing WC, et al. High dose quetiapine in treatment-refractory schizophrenia. *Schizophrenia Res* 2005;**73**:373–5.

333. Glazer WM, Morgenstein H, Pultz J, et al. Incidence of persistent tardive dyskinesia may be lower with quetiapine treatment than previously reported with typical antipsychotics in patients with psychoses. Presented at American College of Neuropsychopharmacology, Acapulco, Mexico, December 1999.

334. Brecher M, Rak IM, Melvin K, et al. The long-term effects on quetiapine (seroquel) monotherapy on weight in patients with schizophrenia. *Int J Psychiat Clin Practice* 2001;**4**:287–91.

335. Sernyak MJ, Leslie DL, Alarcon RD, et al. Association of diabetes mellitus with use of atypical neuroleptics in the treatment of schizophrenia. *Am J Psychiat* 2002;**159**:561–6.

336. Deutschman DA, Deutschman D. High dose ziprasidone: efficacy and tolerability in clinical practice. *Schizophrenia Bull* 2005;**31**(2):480.

337. Potkin SG, Cooper SJ. Ziprasidone and zotepine: clinical experience and use in schizophrenia and mood disorders. In: Buckley PF, Waddington JL, editors. *The New Drug Therapies in Clinical Practice*. Oxford: Arnold, 2000.

338. Keck P, Buffenstein A, Ferguson J, et al. Ziprasidone Study Group. Ziprasidone 40 mg and 20 mg/day in the acute exacerbation of schizophrenia, and schizoaffective disorder: a 4 week placebo controlled trial. *Psychopharmacology* 1998;**140**:173–84.

339. Loebel A, Siu C, Romano S. Improvements in prosocial functioning after a switch to ziprasidone treatment. *CNS Spectrum* 2004;**9**:357–64.

340. Brook Slacy JW, Gunn KP for the Ziprasidone IM Study Group. Intramuscular ziprasidone compared with intramuscular haloperidol in the treatment of acute psychosis. *J Clin Psychiat* 2000;**61**:933–41.

341. Weiden PJ, Simpson GM, Potkin SG, et al. Effectiveness of switching to ziprasidone for stable but symptomatic outpatients with schizophrenia. *J Clin Psychiat* 2003;**64**:580–8.

342. Weiden P, et al. Switching to ziprasidone reduces weight gain. Presentation at American Psychiatric Association Annual Meeting, May 2004, New York.

343. Simpson GM, Glick ID, Weiden PJ, et al. Randomized, controlled, double-blind multicenter comparison of the efficacy and tolerability of ziprasidone and olanzapine in acutely ill inpatients with schizophrenia or schizoaffective disorder. *Am J Psychiatr* 2004;**161**(10):1837–47.

344. Harrigan EP, Micelli JJ, Anziano R, et al. A randomized evaluation of the effects of six antipsychotic agents on Q_{tc}, in the absence and presence of metabolic inhibition. *J Clin Psychopharmacol* 2004;**24**:62–9.

345. Stahl SM. Dopamine system stabilizers, aripiprazole, and the next generation of antipsychotics: "goldilocks" actions at dopamine receptors. *J Clin Psychiat* 2001;**62**:841–2.

346. Stahl SM. Dopamine system stabilizers, aripiprazole, and the next generation of antipsychotics: illustrating their mechanism of action. *J Clin Psychiat* 2001;**62**:923–4.

347. Jordan S, Koprivica V, Chen R, et al. The antipsychotic aripiprazole is a potent, partial agonist at the human 5HT (1A) receptor. *Eur J Pharmacol* 2002;**441**:137–40.

348. McQuade R, Burris K, Jordan S, et al. Aripiprazole: a dopamine–serotonin stabilizer. *Int J Neuropsychopharmacol* 2002;**5**:S176.

349. Kane JM, Carson WH, Saha AR, et al. Efficacy and safety of aripiprazole and haloperidol versus placebo in patients with schizophrenia and schizoaffective disorder. *J Clin Psychiat* 2002;**63**:763–71.

350. Gupta S, Masand P. Aripiprazole: review of its pharmacology and therapeutic use in psychiatric disorders. *Ann Clin Psychiat* 2004;**16**(3):155–66.

351. Potkin SG, Saha AT, Kujawa MJ, et al. Aripiprazole, an antipsychotic with a novel mechanism of action and risperidone vs placebo in patients with schizophrenia and schizoaffective disorder. *Arch Gen Psychiat* 2003;**60**:681–90.

352. McQuade RD, Stock E, Marcus R, et al. A comparison of weight change during treatment with olanzapine or aripiprazole: results from a randomized, double-blind study. *J Clin Psychiat* 2004;**65**(Suppl 18):47–56.

353. Daniel D, et al. Intramuscular aripiprazole in acutely agitated psychotic patients. Presentation at the Annual Meeting of the American Psychiatric Association 2004, New York.

354. Saha AR, Brown D, McEvoy J, et al. Tolerability and efficacy of aripiprazole in patients with first episode schizophrenia: an open-labelled pilot study. *Schizophrenia Res* 2004;**67**:158.

355. Kasper S, Lerman MN, McQuade RD, et al. Efficacy and safety of aripiprazole vs. haloperidol for long-term maintenance treatment following acute relapse of schizophrenia. *Int J Neuropsychopharmacol* 2003;**6**(4):325–37.

356. Kane J, Carson WH, Kujawa M, et al. Aripiprazole in treatment-resistant schizophrenia: a 6 week double blind comparison study versus perphenazine. *Schizophrenia Res* 2004;**67**:155.

357. Casey DE, Carson WH, Saha AR, et al. on behalf of the Aripiprazole Study Group. Switching patients to aripiprazole from other antipsychotic agents: a multicenter randomized study. *Psychopharmacology* 2003;**166**:391–9.

358. Buckley PF, Naber D. Quetiapine and sertindole: clinical use and experience. In: Buckley PF, Waddington JL, editors. *Schizophrenia and Mood Disorders; The New Drug Therapies in Clinical Practice*. London: Arnold Publications, 2000.

359. Kane JM, Tamminga C. Sertindole (serdolect): preclinical and clinical findings of a new atypical antipsychotic. *Expert Opin Invest Drugs* 1997;**6**:1729–41.

360a. Zimbroff DL, Kane JM, Tamminga C, et al. Controlled dose–response study of sertindole and haloperidol in the treatment of schizophrenia. *Am J Psychiat* 1997;**154**:782–91.

360b. Azorin J, Strub N, Loft H. A double-blind, controlled study of sertindole versus risperidone in the treatment of moderate-to-severe schizophrenia. *Intern Clin Psychopharm* 2006;**21**:49–56.

361. Kasper S, Qunier S, Pezawas L. A review of the risk–benefit profile of sertindole. *Int J Psychiat Clin Pract* 1998;**2**:S59–S64.

362. Glassman AH, Bigger JT. Antipsychotic drugs: prolonged qtc interval, torsades de pointes, and sudden death. *Am J Psychiat* 2001;**158**:1774–82.

363a. Lindstrom E, Farde L, Eberhard J, et al. Qtc prolongation and antipsychotic drug treatments: focus on sertindole. *Int J Neuropsychopharmacol* 2005;**8**(4):615–29.

363b. Lis S, Krieger S, Gallhofer B, et al. Sertindole is superior to haloperidol in cognitive performance in patients with schizophrenia: a comparative study. Poster presented at ECNP. Prague, 20–24 September 2003.

364. Colonna L, Saleem P, Dondey-Nouvel P, et al. and the Amisulpiride Study Group. Long term safety and efficacy of amisulpiride in subchronic or chronic schizophrenia. *Int Clin Psychopharmacol* 2000;**15**:13–22.

365. Leucth S, Pitschel-Walz G, Engel RR, et al. Amisulpiride, an unusual 'atypical' antipsychotic: a meta-analysis on randomised controlled trials. *Am J Psychiat* 2002;**159**:180–90.

366. Cooper SJ, Tweed J, Raniwalla J, et al. A placebo controlled comparison of zotepine versus chlorpromazine in patients with acute exacerbation of schizophrenia. *Acta Psychiat Scand* 2000;**101**:218–25.

367. Shiloh R, Zemishlany Z, Aizenberg D, et al. Sulpiride augmentation in people with schizophrenia partially responsive to clozapine: a double-blind, placebo controlled study. *Br J Psychiat* 1997;**171**:569–73.

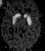
368. Goff DC, Freudenreich O. Focus on polypharmacy in schizophrenia: does anyone truly benefit? *Int J Neuropsychopharmacol* 2004;**7**(2):109–11.

369. Zoccali R, Muscatello MR, Cedro C, et al. The effect of mirtazapine augmentation of clozapine in the treatment of negative symptoms of schizophrenia: a double-blind, placebo-controlled study. *Int Clin Psychopharmacol* 2004;**19**(2):71–6.

370. Kremer I, Vass A, Gorlick I, et al. Placebo-controlled trial of lamotrigine added to conventional and atypical antipsychotics in schizophrenia. *Biol Psychiat* 2004;**156**:441–6.

371. McIntosh AM, Semple D, Tasker K, et al. Transcranial magnetic stimulation for auditory hallucinations in schizophrenia. *Psychiat Res* 2004;**127**(1–2):9–17.

372. Chanpattana W, Kramer BA. Acute and maintenance ECT with flupenthixol in refractory schizophrenia: sustained improvements in psychopathology, quality of life, and social outcomes. *Schizophrenia Res* 2003;**63**(1–2):189–93.

373. Lauriello J, Bustillo J, Keith SJ. A critical review of research on psychosocial treatment of schizophrenia. *Biol Psychiat* 1999;**46**:1409–17.

374. Bustillo J, Lauriello J, Horan W, et al. The psychosocial treatment of schizophrenia: an update. *Am J Psychiat* 2001;**158**:163–75.

375. Fenton WS. Evolving perspectives on individual psychotherapy for schizophrenia. *Schizophrenia Bull* 2000;**26**:47–72.

376. Hogarty G, Kornblith SJ, Greenwald D, et al. Three year trials of personal therapy among schizophrenic patients living with or independent of family. *Am J Psychiat* 1997;**154**:1504–13.

377. Hogarty G, Flesher S, Ulrich R. Cognitive enhancement therapy for schizophrenia: results of a 2-year randomized trial on cognition and behavior. *Arch Gen Psychiat* 2004;**61**:866–76.

378. Garety P, Fowler D, Kuipers E. Cognitive-behavioral therapy for medication resistant symptoms. *Schizophrenia Bull* 2000;**26**:73–86.

379. Dickerson F. Cognitive behavioral psychotherapy for schizophrenia: a review of recent empirical studies. *Schizophrenia Res* 2000;**43**:71–90.

380. Sensky T, Turkington D, Kingdon D, et al. A randomized controlled trial of cognitive behavioral therapy for persistent symptoms in schizophrenia resistant to medication. *Arch Gen Psychiat* 2000;**57**:165–72.

381. Haddock G, Morrison AP, Hopkins R, et al. Individual cognitive behavioural interventions in early psychosis. *Br J Psychiat* 1998;**172**(Suppl 33):101–6.

382. Kemp RA, Kirov G, Everitt B, et al. Randomised controlled trial of compliance therapy; 18 month follow up. *Br J Psychiat* 1998;**172**:413–9.

383. Dixon L, Adams C, Lucksted A. Update on the family psychoeducation of schizophrenia. *Schizophrenia Bull* 2000;**26**:5–20.

384. Heinssen RK, Liberman RP, Kopelowicz A. Psychosocial skills training for schizophrenia: lessons from the laboratory. *Schizophrenia Bull* 2000;**26**:21–46.

385. Green MF. Neurocognition and functional outcome. *Schizophrenia Bull* 2000;**26**:119–36.

386. Harvey PD, Green MF, Keefe RS, et al. Cognitive functioning in schizophrenia: a consensus statement on its role in the definition and evaluation of effective treatments for the illness. *J Clin Psychiat* 2004;**65**(3):361–72.

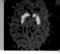

387. Thornicroft G, Sczumkler G. *A Textbook of Community Psychiatry*. Oxford: Oxford University Press, 2001.

388. Simmonds S, Coid J, Joseph P, et al. Community mental health team management in severe mental illness: a systematic review. *Br J Psychiat* 2001;**178**:497–502.

389. Gray R, Wykes T, Edmonds M, et al. Effect of a medication management training package for nurses on clinical outcomes for patients with schizophrenia: cluster randomised controlled trial. *Br J Psychiat* 2004;**185**:157–62.

390. Lehman AF, Goldberg R, Dixon LB, et al. Improving employment outcomes for persons with severe mental illness. *Arch Gen Psychiat* 2002;**59**:165–72.

391. Bell M, Bryson G, Greig T, et al. Neurocognitive enhancement therapy with work therapy. *Arch Gen Psychiat* 2001;**58**:763–8.

392. Kurtz MM, Moberg PJ, Gur RC, Gur RE. Results from randomized, controlled trials of the effects of cognitive remediation on neurocognitive deficits in patients with schizophrenia. *Psychol Med* 2004;**34**(3):569–70.

393. President's New Freedom Commission. *Transforming America's Mental Health System*, 2003.

394. Hughes DH, Kleepies PM. Treating aggression in the psychiatric emergency service. *J Clin Psychiat* 2003;**64**(4):10–5.

395. Currier GW, Allen MH, Bunney EB, et al. Updated treatment algorithm. *J Emerg Med* 2004;**4**:525–6.

396. Monahan J, Redlich AD, Swanson J, et al. Use of leverage to improve adherence to psychiatric treatment in the community. *Psychiat Serv* 2005;**56**:37–44.

397. Lieberman JA, Perkins D, Belger A, et al. The early stages of schizophrenia: speculations on the pathogensis, pathophysiology, and therapeutic approaches. *Biol Psychiat* 2001;**50**:884–97.

398. Tran PV, Hamilton SH, Kuntz AJ, et al. Double-blind comparison of olanzapine vs risperidone in the treatment of schizophrenia and other psychotic disorders. *J Clin Psychopharmacol* 1997;**17**:407–18.

399. Bon-Choon H, Miller D, Nopoulos P, et al. A comparative effectiveness study of risperidone and olanzapine in the treatment of schizophrenia. *J Clin Psychiat* 1999;**60**:658–63.

400. Conley RB, Mahmoud R. A randomized double blind study of risperidone and olanzapine in the treatment of schizophrenia or schizoaffective disorder. *Am J Psychiat* 2001;**158**:1759–63.

401. Breier A, Kane JM, Berg PH, Thakore DN, et al. Olanzapine versus ziprasidone: results of the 28-week double-blind study in patients with schizophrenia. *Am J Psychiat* 2005, in press.

402. Zhong K, Harvey P, Brecher M. A randomized, double-blind study of quetiapine and risperidone in the treatment of schizophrenia. *Schizophrenia Bull* 2005;**31**(2):508.

403. Rupnow MF, Stahl S, Greenspan A, et al. Use and cost of polypharmacy in schizophrenia: data from a randomized, double-blind study of risperidone and quetiapine. *Schizophrenia Bull* 2005;**31**(2):550.

404. Addington DE, Pantelis C, Dineen M, et al. Efficacy and tolerability of ziprasidone versus risperidone in patients with acute exacerbation of schizophrenia or schizoaffective disorder: an 8-week, double-blind, multicenter trial. *J Clin Psychiat* 2004;**65**:1624–33.

405. Voruganti L, Cortese L, Oyewumi L, et al. Comparative evaluation of conventional and novel antipsychotic drugs with reference to their subjective tolerability, side-effect profile and impact on quality of life. *Schizophrenia Res* 2000;**43**:135–45.

406. Blackburn G. Weight gain and antipsychotic medications. *J Clin Psychiat* 2000;**61**:36–42.

407. Welch R, Chue P. Antipsychotic agents and QT changes. *J Psychiat Neurosci* 2000;**25**:154–60.

408. Reilly M, Ayis S, Ferrier I, et al. QTc-interval abnormalities and psychotropic drug therapy in psychiatric patients. *Lancet* 2000;**355**:1048–52.

409. Masellis M, Basile V, Ozdemir V, et al. Pharmacogenetics of antipsychotic treatment: lessons learned from clozapine. *Biol Psychiat* 2000;**47**:252–66.

410. Fichtner CG, Luchins DJ, Malan RD, et al. Real-world pharmaco-therapy with novel antipsychotics. *J Pract Psychiat Behav Health* 1999;**5**:37–43.

411. Weiden PJ, Casey DE. "Polypharmacy": combining antipsychotic medications in the treatment of schizophrenia. *J Pract Psychiat Behav Health* 1999;**5**:229–33.

412. Kinon BJ, Burson BR, Gilmore JA, et al. Strategies for switching from conventional antipsychotic drugs or risperidone to olanzapine. *J Clin Psychiat* 2000;**61**:833–40.

413. Wirshing DA, Marshall BD, Green MF, et al. Risperidone in treatment-refractory schizophrenia. *Am J Psychiat* 1999;**156**:1374–9.

414. Breier A, Hamilton SH. Comparative efficacy of olanzapine and haloperidol for patients with treatment resistant schizophrenia. *Biol Psychiat* 1999;**45**:403–11.

415. Conley RR, Tamminga CA, Kelly DL, et al. Treatment-resistant schizophrenic patients respond to clozapine after olanzapine non-response. *Biol Psychiat* 1999;**46**:73–7.

416. Heresco-Levy U, Ermilov M, Lichtenberg P, Bar G, Javitt DC. High-dose glycine added to olanzapine and risperidone for the treatment of schizophrenia. *Biol Psychiat* 2004;**55**(2):165–71.

417. Siris SG, Addington D, Azorin JM, et al. Depression and management in the USA. *Schizophrenia Res* 2001;**47**:185–97.

418. Roy A, Thompson R, Kennedy S. Depression in chronic schizophrenia. *Br J Psychiat* 1983;**142**:465–70.

419. Siris SG. Depression in schizophrenia: perspective in the era of atypical antipsychotic agents. *Am J Psychiat* 2000;**157**:1379–89.

420. Green AI, Canuso CM, Brenner MJ, et al. Detection and management of comorbidity in patients with schizophrenia. *Psychiat Clin North Am* 2003;**26**:115–39.

421. Buckley PF, Noffsinger S, Smith DA, et al. Treatment of the psychotic patient who is violent. *Psychiat Clin North Am* 2003;**26**(1):231–72.

422. Taylor PJ, Estroff S. Schizophrenia and the risk of violence. In: Hirsch SR, Weinberger DR, editors. *Schizophrenia*, 2nd ed. Oxford: Blackwell Science, 2003; pp. 163–83.

423. Hughes DH, Kleespies PM. Treating aggression in the psychiatric emergency service. *J Clin Psychiat* 2003;**64**(Suppl 4):10–5.

424. Walsh E, Buchanan A, Fahy T. Violence and schizophrenia: examining the evidence. *Br J Psychiat* 2002;**180**:490–5.

425. Swartz M, Swenson J, Hiday V, et al. Randomized, controlled trial of out-patient commitment in North Carolina. *Psych Services* 2001;**52**:325–9.

426. Drake RE, Mueser KT. Psychosocial approaches to dual diagnosis. *Schizophrenia Bull* 2000;**26**:105–18.

427. Barraclough C, Haddock G, Tarrier N, et al. Randomized controlled trial of motivational interviewing, cognitive behavioral therapy, and family intervention for patients with comorbid schizophrenia and substance use disorders. *Am J Psychiat* 2001;**158**:1706–13.

428. Buckley PF. Treatment of substance abuse in schizophrenia. *J Clin Psychiat* 1998;**59**:26–30.

429. Berman I, Berman SM, Lengua JA, et al. Obsessive and compulsive symptoms in chronic schizophrenia. *Comp Psychiat* 1995;**36**:6–10.

430. Conley RB. New drugs on the horizon. In: Buckley PF, Waddington JL, editors. *Schizophrenia and Mood Disorders: The New Drug Therapies in Clinical Practice*. Oxford: Arnold, 2001.

431. Mahadik SP, Evans DR. Is schizophrenia a metabolic brain disorder? Membrane phospholipid dysregulation and its therapeutic implications. *Psychiat Clin North Am* 2003;**26**:85–102.

432. Theisen FM, Hinney A, Bromel T, et al. Lack of association between the -759C/T polymorphism of the 5-HT2C receptor gene and clozapine-induced weight gain among German schizophrenic individuals. *Psychiat Genet* 2004;**14**(3):139–42.

433. Young RM, Lawford BR, Barnes M, et al. Prolactin levels in antipsychotic treatment of patients with schizophrenia carrying the DRD2*A1 allele. *Br J Psychiat* 2004;**185**:147–51.

434. Abdi Z, Sharma T. Social cognition and its neural correlates in schizophrenia and autism. *CNS Spectrum* 2004;**9**(5):335–43.

435. Bellack AS, Schooler NR, Marder SR, et al. Do clozapine and risperidone affect social competence and problem solving? *Am J Psychiat* 2004;**161**(2):364–7.

436. Geyer MA, Tamminga CA. Measurment and treatment research to improve cognition in schizophrenia: neuropharmacological aspects. *Psychopharmacology* 2004;**174**(1):1–2.

437. Druss BG, Rohrbaugh RM, Levinson CM, et al. Integrated medical care for patients with serious psychiatric illness. *Arch Gen Psychiat* 2001;**58**:861–8.

438. Drake R, Mueser K, Torrey W, et al. Evidence-based treatment of schizophrenia. *Curr Psychiat Rep* 2000;**2**:393–7.

439. Carpenter WT. Evidence-based treatment for first-episode schizophrenia? *Am J Psychiat* 2001;**158**:1771–3.

Index

Note: As schizophrenia is the subject of the book, all index entries refer to schizophrenia unless otherwise indicated. Page numbers in *italics* refer to figures and/or tables; those followed by (cs) refer to case studies.

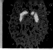

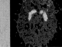

DATE DUE

DEC 1 8 2006	
APR 0 3 2007	DEC 1 3 2010
OCT 0 3 2007	
	NOV 0 1 2011
OCT 2 0 2008	DEC 0 9 2011
FEB 1 2 2009	FEB 2 4 2012
JUL 0 2 2009	APR 1 4 2016 MAY 9 2012
NOV 1 4 2009	APR 3 0 OCT 0 3 2012
APR 2 0 2010	
OCT 0 4 2010	
DEC 0 7 2013	APR 2 8 2014